the essentials in
echocardiography

THE TARDIEU SERIES

the essentials in echocardiography

I

J.-L. LAURENCEAU MD, PH D
Assistant Professor Laval University
and Institut de Cardiologie de Québec
Echocardiographic Laboratory
• Hôpital de la Salpêtrière
• CMC de la Porte de Choisy
Paris

M.-C. MALERGUE MD
Assistant Professor Paris University
Echocardiographic Laboratory
• Hôpital Bichat
• CMC de la Porte de Choisy
Paris

Bernard TARDIEU
Medical Illustrator

Foreword by A.J. Tajik
Mayo Clinic, Rochester, Minn.

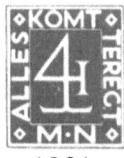

1981
MARTINUS NIJHOFF PUBLISHERS
THE HAGUE / BOSTON / LONDON

Distributors :

for the United States and Canada

Kluwer Boston, Inc.
190 Old Derby Street
Hingham, MA 02043
USA

for all other countries

Kluwer Academic Publishers Group
Distribution Center
P.O. Box 322
3300 AH Dordrecht
The Netherlands

This volume is listed in the Library of Congress Cataloging in Publication Data

ISBN-13: 978-90-247-2482-6   e-ISBN-13: 978-94-009-8285-7
DOI: 10.1007/ 978-94-009-8285-7

FOREWORD

Echocardiography has become an essential tool for good practice of cardiology. Introduction of 2-D echocardiography has opened a new era of cardiac imaging and investigation. The rapid progress in the field of echocardiography has created an extreme need, now more than ever, for a practical book which is concise, yet complete, well illustrated with good quality tracings and which provides the latest information on the state of the art of combined M-Mode and 2-D) echocardiography. In this book « The Essentials in Echocardiography » Drs. Laurenceau and Malergue have done an excellent job of accomplishing above goals as they discuss the basics of ultrasound, normal examination, and features of various diseases of the heart. The format of presentation, the quality of illustrations and the clarity of discussion point to the thorough and broad echographic experience of these authors. By sharing their experience with us in the form of this well-conceived book, they have done the field of echocardiography a great service.

A. J. TAJIK, M.D. FACC
Consultant in Cardiovascular Diseases
and Pediatric Cardiology
Director of Echocardiographic Laboratories
Mayo Clinic

TABLE OF CONTENTS

PART II: Congenital heart disease

PREFACE

Although the phenomenon of ultrasound was discovered many years ago, it was only after tests had shown it to have no deleterious effects that it was used as a diagnostic tool in medicine.

Its rapid development in many disciplines, especially cardiology, in the last few years is due to the non-invasive character of ultrasonic examination: it is a painless, easily repeatable and reproduceable, economic investigation, which rapidly makes available a wealth of information which can usually only be obtained by more invasive techniques.

We have felt an increasing need for a practical and well illustrated book (because of the very graphic nature of the method), describing the essentials of echocardiography, with the object of being complete rather than comprehensive. The two forms of echocardiography, M-mode and real time two-dimensional echocardiography, are presented in an integrated fashion. The present volume contains a review of the physics of ultrasound and an explanation of the different modes of recording followed by an analysis of the normal echocardiographic appearances. This is followed by a discussion of the findings in most of the congenital cardiac malformations.

A second volume will be given over to the study of acquired heart disease (valvular, myocardial and pericardial disease and cardiac tumours). The changes observed in the principal arrhythmias and the cardiac manifestations of certain collagen diseases are also treated.

This book is aimed at physicians, students and technicians wishing to learn echocardiography, but it may also be of use to those already initiated in the technique who wish to perfect their understanding, especially of the interpretation of the two-dimensional examination. Each condition is described from the anatomical and echocardiographic point of view, with a discussion on the relative value of each diagnostic sign.

The echocardiogrammes were recorded by the authors in three laboratories. Those marked with an asterisk come from Doctor Kalmanson's department, (Fondation Ophthalmologique Rothschild - Paris) and were recorded on an ATL III instrument. We take this opportunity of expressing our thanks for his cooperation. The other documents were recorded either at the Cardiological Institute of Quebec (Smith Kline instrument) or at the Centre Médico-chirurgical de la Porte de Choisy, Paris (Roche RT 400 and Irex II).

It was at Quebec that we started practicing echocardiography and we would particularly like to thank Doctors A. Moisan, J.G. Dumesnil and S. Gagné, as well as Mrs A. April and Mr J. Beauchemin for their help and encouragement at that time.

We also thank the staff of the Centre Médico-chirurgical de la Porte de Choisy and Doctors J. Aigueperse, Y. Lecompte, G. Lemoine, J. Temkine, as well as Mme E. Regnier and Mr J.F. Arlene for their collaboration in the writing of this book.

Our thanks also go to our mentors, Professors Y. Bouvrain, Y. Grosgogeat and R. Tricot, as well as to their assistants.

COMMON ABBREVIATIONS

Ao: Aorta
C.S.: coronary sinus
I.A.S.: inter atrial septum
I.V.C.: inferior vena cava
I.V.S.: interventricular septum
L.A.: left atrium
L.A.O.: left anterior oblique
L.V.: left ventricle
L.V.W.: left ventricle wall
A.L.W.: anterolateral wall
A.W.: anterior wall
L.W.: lateral wall
P.W.: posterior wall
M. or M.V.: mitral valve
A.M.L.: anterior mitral leaflet
P.M.L.: posterior mitral leaflet
P.A.: pulmonary artery
P. or P.V.: Pulmonary valve
P. Vn: pulmonary vein
R.A.: right atrium
R.A.O.: right anterior oblique
R.V.: right ventricle
R.V.O.T.: right ventricle outflow tract
T. or T.V.: tricuspid valve
A.T.L.: anterior tricuspid leaflet
P.T.L.: posterior tricuspid leaflet
S.T.L.: septal tricuspid leaflet
Th Ao: Thoracic Aorta
T.M.: Time Motion
2D: Two Dimensional

PART I

CHAPTER 1

PHYSICS OF ULTRASOUND AND INSTRUMENTATION

1.1. HISTORY OF ECHOCARDIOGRAPHY

Although X-Rays were used in medical diagnosis soon after their discovery, the application of diagnostic ultrasound was much more progressive. Experimental studies in man were very carefully conducted to eliminate the possibility of side effects similar to those of ionising radiations[122].

The first practical use of ultrasound was the asdic or sonar detection of submarines (Langevin[115]). This property was fully exploited for military objectives, mainly during the Second World War. More pacific uses were blocked because of the classified nature of these usages until the end of the war. Shortly afterwards, Firestone[56] published a study of flaw detection in metals, using an ex-military ultrasonoscope.

The first medical application of ultrasound dates back to the early 1950's (Howry[94], Wild[234], Keidel[102]). In 1954, two Swedes, Edler and Hertz[47], were the first to visualise cardiac structures in motion. This was the beginning of echocardiography: they developed the technique of M mode recording, displaying the echos on an oscilloscope with respect to time. The technical limitations of their instrument only allowed detection of echos reflected by the pericardium, the most echogenic cardiac structure. After improving the equipment, Edler, in 1961[49] showed how the heart valves and walls could be indentified and also described the appearances of mitral and aortic stenosis, left atrial tumours and pericardial effusions. Echocardiography was introduced to the United States in 1963, by Reid. Since then, the technique has been greatly expanded, and the number of medical publications on this subject has increased accordingly[97].

Some workers perfected methods of visualising the cardiac cavities (Gramiak[75], 1969), whilst others used the Doppler effect to study intracardiac blood flow[95] [99] [100].

Finally, the last few years have seen the development of a new generation of instruments giving real-time, cross-sectional images of the heart by mechanical or electronic scanning; they have opened up a new field, that of two-dimensional echocardiography[12] [79] [220], (Bom, Griffith, Von Ramm).

1.2. PHYSICAL PROPERTIES OF ULTRASOUND[4] [20] [54] [73] [221]

A certain knowledge of the physical properties of ultrasound is necessary to fully understand echocardiography.

1.2.1. Definitions

Sound is the transmission of energy in the form of vibration *(frequency)* of particles in a particular medium. *Frequency* is the number of compressions or rarefactions (fig. 1-1) per second. This is expressed in cycles per second or Hertz (Hz). The audible range of human ear varies from 30-50 Hz to 15 000 Hz.

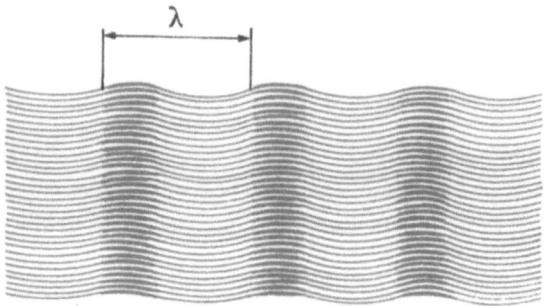

Fig. 1-1 Sound: series of compressions and expansions

By definition, ultrasound has a frequency greater than 20 000 Hz, which means that it is above the range of human audibility. The frequencies used in cardiology range from one million Hz (1 MHz) to 7 MHz, with intensities of less than 100 milliwatts per cm^2.

The wave length (λ) is the distance between two successive cycles. The velocity represents the speed with which the sound waves travel through a given medium. As all sound waves in a given beam have the same velocity, the distance travelled by the ultrasound per unit of time is equal to the product of their frequency and wavelength:

$$c = \lambda\ f \qquad \begin{array}{ll} c & \textbf{velocity of sound in the medium} \\ \lambda & \textbf{wavelength} \\ f & \textbf{frequency in Hz} \end{array}$$

The soft tissues of the human body may be likened to a homogenous conductor, such as normal saline, in which the propagation of ultrasound is relatively constant (1 540 m/sec). On the other hand, the velocity is much higher in bone (3 380 m/sec), and much lower in air (354 m/sec). These two media strongly absorb ultrasound, and are therefore very poor conductors[73].

1.2.2. Acoustic Impedance

This term describes the acoustic properties of a medium: by definition, the *acoustic impedance* (Z) is the product of the density of the medium (P) and the velocity of sound in the medium (C): Z = PC.

The surface of separation between two media of different accoustic impedance is called an *acoustic interface*. At each acoustic interface, part of the ultrasound beam is reflected and part is refracted (fig. 1-2): the greater is the difference of acoustic impedance between two media (acoustic mismatch), the greater the amount of sound is reflected.

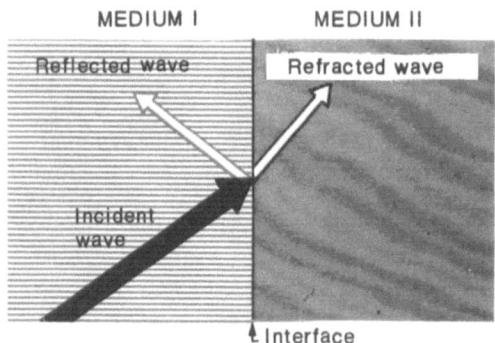

Fig. 1-2 Refraction and reflection at an interface separating two media of different acoustic impedance

1.2.3. Resolution and penetration

When a frequency of 2,25 MHz is used (the frequency normally used in adult echocardiography), a wavelenght of the ultrasonic beam of 0,7 mm is obtained: $\lambda = \dfrac{C}{F}$. When the frequency is doubled (a value normally used in paediatric echocardiography), the wavelength is halved. Theoretically, the distance between two structures must be greater than a quarter of the wavelength for two separate echos to be identified *(resolution)*. In practice, it is difficult to obtain a better resolution than one wavelength: therefore, the higher the frequency is, the higher the resolution is. However, at high frequencies, greater amounts of ultrasound are reflected by proximal tissues with a rapid fall-off of energy. As a result, the depth of penetration of the ultrasound beam is reduced and the distal echos are attenuated.

To summarise, the higher the frequency and the shorter the wavelength the better is the resolution; however, the ultrasound beam loses its energy of penetration and deep-lying structures cannot be recorded.

All ultrasonic probes currently used in diagnostic ultrasound are composed of piezo-electric crystals. Piezo-electricity is the property of certain substances to change the mechanical energy of deformation into electric energy and vice versa.

Commercial transducers use ceramics as piezo-electric elements. The most commonly used are baryum titanate and lead zinconate titanate. Behind the piezo-electric element is some backing material which absorbs the ultrasound directed backwards, and improves the shape of the forward beam (fig. 1-3). The echocardiograph acts both as a transmitter and a receiver of ultrasound. It transmits for a very short time, and then "receives" the reflected echos. The duration of the transmission is usually 1/1000 of the reception time and only lasts one microsecond. Therefore, there is an emission each millisecond. This method of acoustic imaging is called pulsed ultrasound.

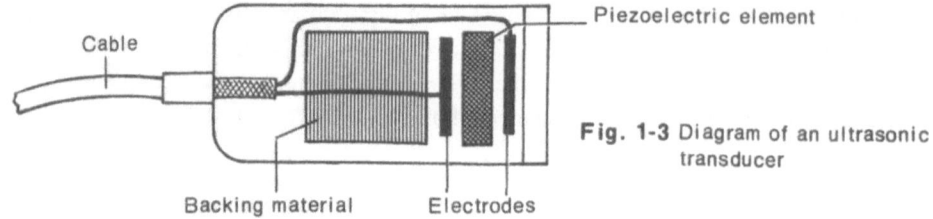

Cable

Piezoelectric element

Fig. 1-3 Diagram of an ultrasonic
transducer

Backing material   Electrodes

1.2.5. Reflection and divergence

The propagation of ultrasound is similar to that of light; the same physical laws apply. The ultrasonic beam must be perpendicular to the structures under study in order to record the reflected echos.

Certain properties of the ultrasonic beam must be appreciated. It remains essentially parallel for a given distance (the near or Fresnel field), and then begins to diverge (the far or Fraunhofer field). The distance, at which the beam begins to diverge, is given by the following formula:

$$d = \frac{R^2}{\lambda}$$

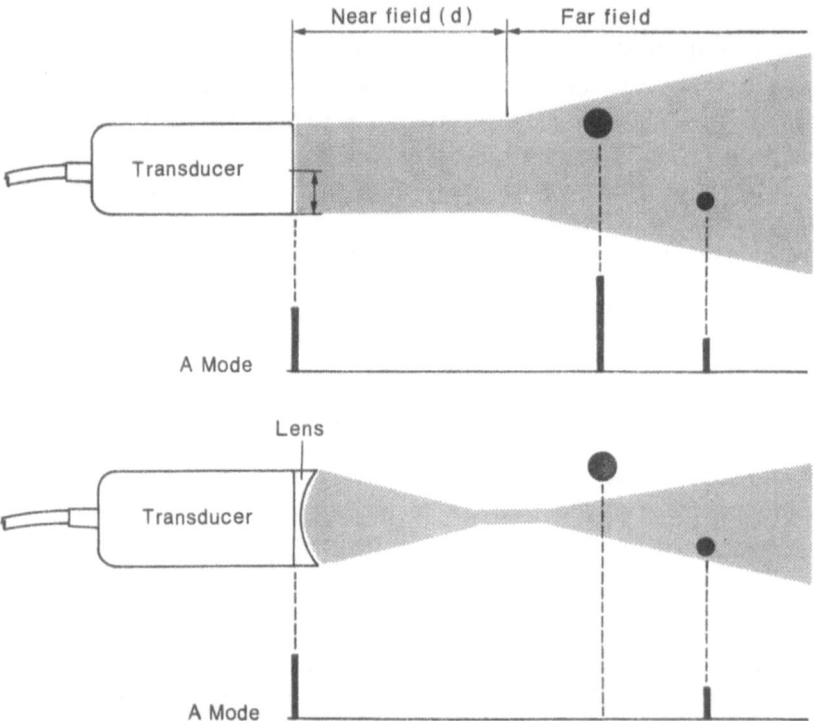

Fig. 1-4 Top: diagram showing the near and far fields without focusing. The two non-aligned objects are recorded on the same ultrasonic axis because of divergence of the beam in the far field
Bottom: improved lateral resolution with an acoustic lens.

1.2.6. Latéral resolution

The ultrasonic beam is as wide as the diameter of the transducer in the near field, but it undergoes divergence in the far field. The beam is therefore not a point source, the diameter of the transducer usually being between 5 and 12 mm. This explains why two structures which are not in line with respect to the transducer, may appear artefactually aligned on the recording (fig. 1-4, *lateral resolution*). This effect is more marked in the distal field.

Acoustic lenses of known focal length (usually 5 to 10 cm), may be used to improve lateral resolution (fig. 1-4).

1.2.7. The Doppler effects[96]

The Doppler effect may be used in diagnostic ultrasonics. When a beam of ultrasound passes through a moving column of blood, there is some back-scattering of energy. The frequency of the reflected signal is modified by the velocity and direction of the blood flow with respect to the incidence of the ultrasonic beam. Movement towards the transducer increases the frequency and movement away decreases the frequency of the reflected signal. This change in frequency is proportional to the velocity of blood flow and the angle between the ultrasound beam and the moving target. When the direction of the blood flow is perpendicular to the beam, its velocity cannot be measured (fig. 1-5). Using pulsed Doppler systems, the Doppler effect may be measured at a given distance from the transducer, so providing information on the velocity and direction of blood flow at a precise location within the thorax.

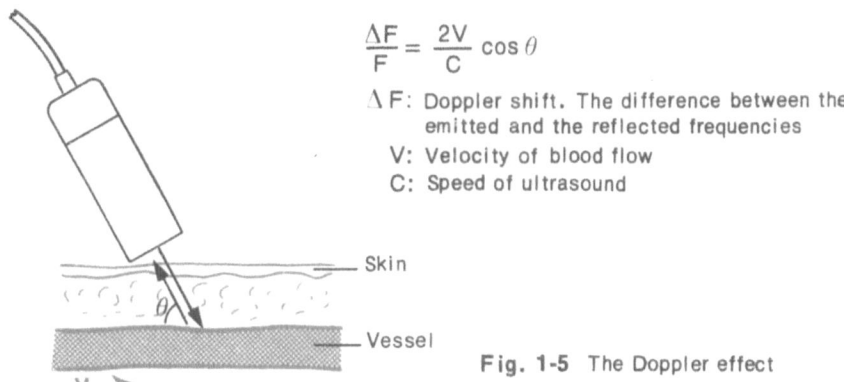

$$\frac{\Delta F}{F} = \frac{2V}{C} \cos \theta$$

ΔF: Doppler shift. The difference between the emitted and the reflected frequencies
V: Velocity of blood flow
C: Speed of ultrasound

Fig. 1-5 The Doppler effect

1.3. INSTRUMENTATION

1.3.1. Uni-directional echocardiographs

A) *Display*

The echocardiograph functions both as a transmitter of pulsed ultrasound, and a receiver of the reflected echos.

There are three modes of display of these echoes: A mode (A = amplitude), B mode (B = brightness), and M mode (M = motion) (fig. 1-6)

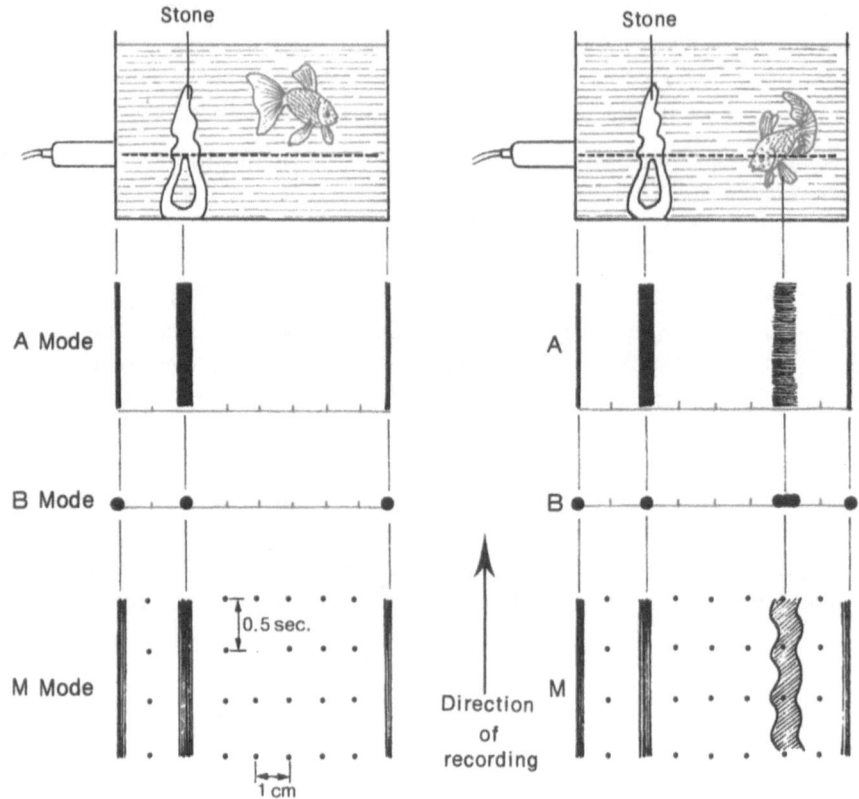

Fig. 1-6 A, B and M modes of acoustic imaging
The immobile object (stone) gives rise to echos at fixed depth whereas the fish reflects echos according to its position which cannot be analysed by A and B modes: time motion display allows interpretation of its movement

— *A mode* displays the reflected echos as vertical spikes on a horizontal base line. The amplitude of each spike varies with the intensity of each reflected echoe, the base line being calibrated for distance. Although little used nowadays, it is very useful for adjusting the various echocardiographic controls.

— *B mode* retains the same horizontal base line, but the reflected echos are displayed as dots rather than spikes. The intensity or brightness of each spot is proportional to the amplitude of the spike. This mode is used for the display of two-dimensional echography, and also for the recording of M mode echocardiograms on strip chart recorders.

— *M mode* is obtained by electronically tracking the B mode on an oscilloscope. The B mode echos are therefore displayed with respect to time and their motion appears as a wavy line: in unidirectional echocardiography, M mode is a method of presenting the different phases of the cardiac cycle, and of recording and analysing them. For convenience, M mode is displayed from left to right on the oscilloscope, the top of the screen corresponding to the position of the transducer.

B) *Controls*

Most M mode echographs have both A mode and M mode display, a fiber optic strip chart recorder and various control knobs. The adjustments (fig. 1-7), which are made on the A mode screen, are of two sorts:

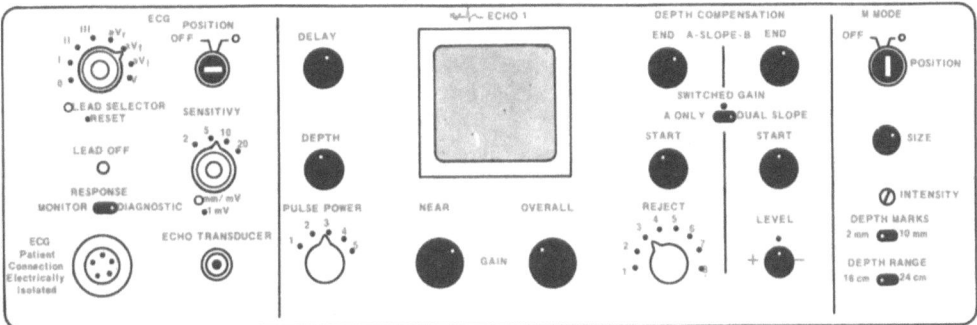

Fig. 1-7   M Mode control module on a commercially available echocardiograph.
The adjustments are made an the A Mode screen. The M Mode display is on a separate screen

a) *Adjustment of the position and size of the Image*

This depends on the size of the heart under study, the depth control having to be widened for children: this avoids reverberations (fig. 1-8) and gives optimal visualisation of cardiac structures. The position control or delay allows the operator to change the position of the image without altering the depth control. This makes room for other physiological signals on the same recording.

b) *Adjustment of the quality and intensity of the image*

This is performed by adjusting the emission and/or by processing the reflected echos by a system of echo enhancement (A mode). The gain-control allows enhancement of the reflected echos without altering the intensity of the pulsed emission.

Ultrasound is attenuated and decreases in intensity as it travels in the tissues, so that echos reflected from deep lying structures are weaker than those reflected from proximal ones: to compensate for this effect, most echographs have a control which allows selective attenuation of near field echos and/or enhancement of far field echos (Time - gain compensation). The

17

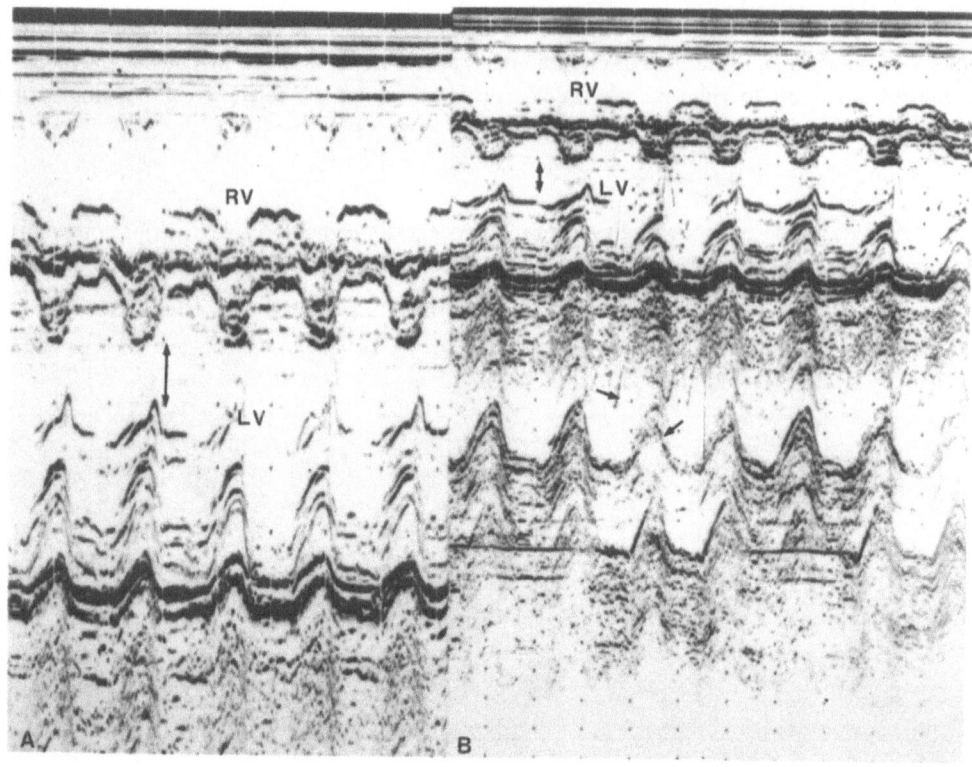

Fig. 1-8 Echocardiogram demonstrating reverberation
A- Correct adjustment of depth control
B- The depth scale is twice as small. Reverberations (➤) probably arising from the mitral valve and left ventricular posterior wall.

compensating mechanism is displayed as a "ramp", the start and slope of which may be adjusted. A separate adjustment (near gain) is used to control the intensity of near field echos. Some echographs have a programmable time-gain control which allows adjustment of the gain for each depth of examination (fig. 1-9).

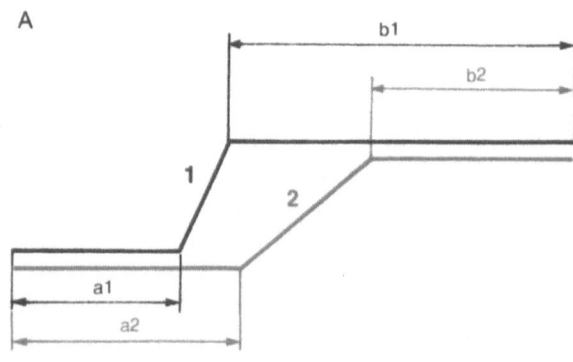

Fig. 1-9 Depth compensation control

A: The usual controle where by the start and slope of a single "ramp" may be adjusted

a1 a2 : near gain

b1 b2 : coarse gain

1 2 : slopes

B

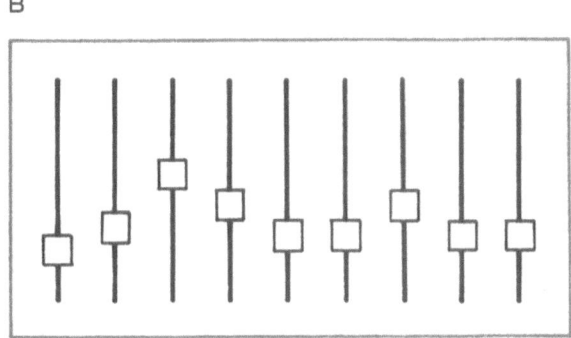

Fig. 1-9

B: Multiple depth
   compensation
   controls

Reject: the reject control is an electronic device which allows elimination of signals of weak intensity at reception, but the threshold should not be too high, otherwise, useful signals may be suppressed.

Damping: this controls the intensity of the ultrasound beam on emission. It is useful for the identification of two closely situated strong echos, such as the epicardo-pericardial complex from the neighbouring structures.

Switch gain: some modern echographs have a control which acts as a continuous damping and allows better definition of the left ventricular posterior wall.

C) *Recording*

Whichever type of recording chosen, it is essential to have a simultaneous ECG (lead DII is generally used). This serves as a chronological marker for echocardiographic events.

In the early days of echocardiography, the only method of recording was by photographing the oscilloscope (usually by Polaroid). This was of limited value because of the relatively small number of cardiac cycles on each oscilloscopic sweep. In recent years, it has become possible to record M mode echocardiography on paper. The recordings may be made at variable paper speeds, 25 or 50 mm/sec for routine recording, 75 or 100 mm/sec for analysis of rapid events.

Several types of recording paper are commercially available: ultraviolet light sensitive and dry silver heat sensitive paper are the two generally used, the essential feature being instantaneous development for immediate control of the quality of the recording.

1.3.2. Two-dimensional Echocardiographs

As M mode echocardiography only gives an image of the heart along a single line with respect to time, many techniques were suggested to visualise dynamic anatomical planes of the heart. Many terms have been proposed to describe these techniques: cross-sectional echocardiography, real time, two-dimensional, multiscan and echotomocardiography...

The principal technique used in two-dimensional echocardiographic recording is compound B scanning. A certain number of lines of B mode are recorded simultaneously on the oscilloscope screen. When viewed together, they produce an image of a section of the heart which varies with the position and angle of the transducer. These images are reproduced at a rate of about 30 per sec, to give a dynamic, real-time scan.

Three different systems are available for two-dimensional echocardiography, but all use video systems for its recording (fig. 1-10).

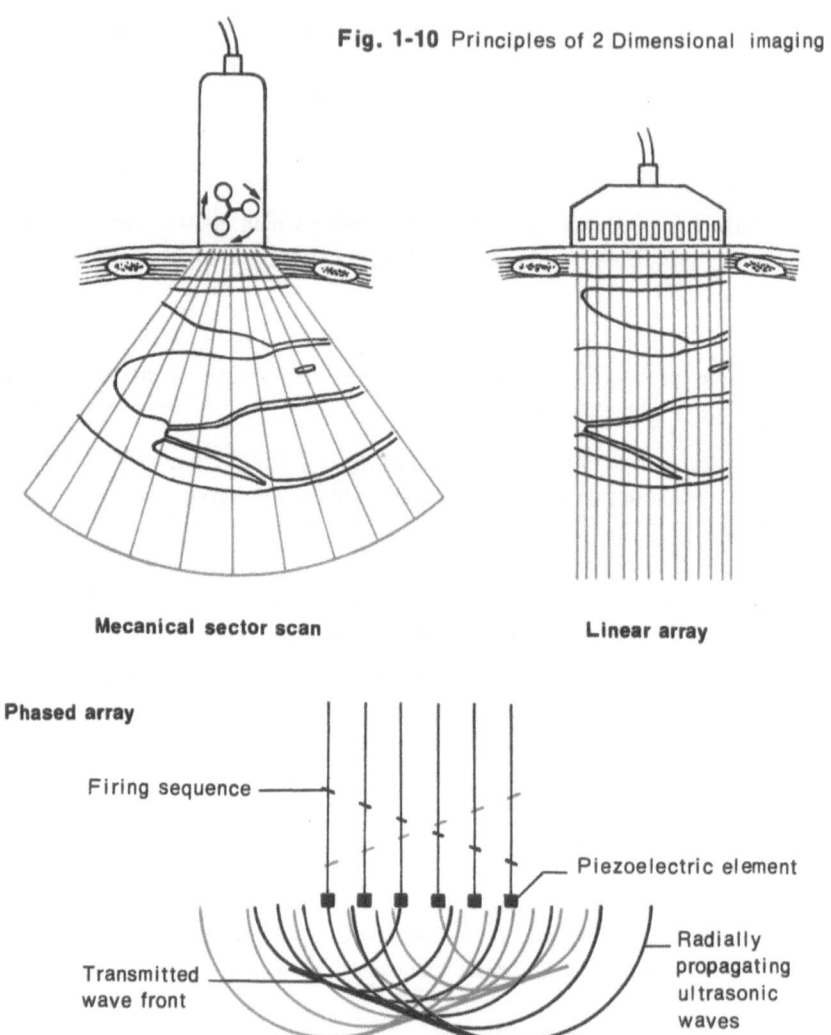

Fig. 1-10 Principles of 2 Dimensional imaging

Mecanical sector scan

Linear array

Phased array

Firing sequence

Piezoelectric element

Transmitted wave front

Radially propagating ultrasonic waves

— *Mechanical transducer*[79]: this is probably the simplest and cheapest system. The image is obtained by a rapid rotation of one or several transducers by an electric motor. The resulting image is displayed as a sector of a circle, with each line of B mode originating at the center.

— *Linear Array Multiscan*[12]: this system comprises a linear array of a number of small ultrasonic elements on the transducer. The elements are activated rapidly in sequence each giving a line of B mode echos. These systems require quite large transducers, which have two practical disadvantages: the transducer crosses the ribs and certain anatomical planes cannot be examined.

— *Phased Array Sector Scan*[220]: this is probably the most sophisticated technique for obtaining two-dimensional images of the heart. The transducer is about 2 cm wide allowing positioning between the ribs; it also employs multiple elements, usually about thirty, which are activated in sequence with an electronically timed delay so that the ultrasonic wave front is at an angle with the transducer.

By changing the sequence of activation, it is possible to sweep the beam through a sector of 80 to 90°. These systems may also be equipped with a variable acoustic, focus.

These echocardiographs are costly but provide high quality echocardiograms. They are continually being perfected, and are probably, the future of echocardiography.

— *Simultaneous M mode:* phased array sector scans have the option of one or two lines of M mode which may be recorded at the same time as the two-dimensional image (fig. 1-11).

M mode coupled with 2D allows the recording of structures which are often difficult to visualise, such as the pulmonary valve; it also offers a method for analysis of echocardiographic events which are too rapid to be studied by 2D.

It is also possible to integrate the sample volume of pulsed Doppler echocardiography on this line of M mode.

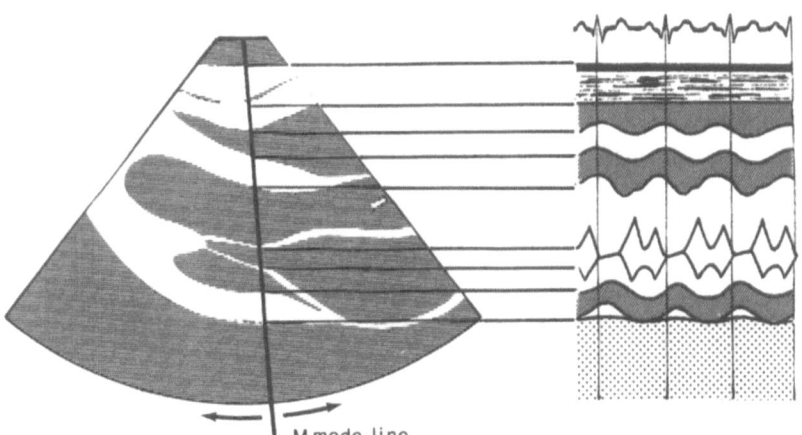

Fig. 1-11
2D and simultaneous M mode echocardiography. The M mode line defines the structures displayed in M mode: in this illustration it is centered on the mitral valve

M mode line

1.3.3. Complementary investigations

— *Phono and pulse recording*

This is recorded simultaneously with M mode, and is useful in the study of the timing of heart sounds with respect to the valvular motion on echo, and also helps in the analysis of the function of prosthetic heart valves. It is essential that these cases are recorded at rapid paper speeds[34] [105].

— Dual echo

This is the simultaneous recording of two M mode echocardiograms, a useful technique for measuring the isovolumetric periods[137].

— Other parameters

Respiration, pressure curves, Doppler, etc.[80]

— Pharmacodynamic and physiological tests

Valsalva manœuver, isometric or isotonic exercise tests, changing position, amyl nitrite, glyceryl trinitrate, etc.[106] [132] [153].

— Contrast echocardiography

The injection of certain echogenic substances allow visualisation of the cardiac cavities[75]. The most commonly used are normal saline, dextrose and indocyanine green, although reinjection of the patients own blood may also be used[52] [182] [199]. The mechanism of this phenomenon remains controversial: cavitation and turbulence, different acoustic impedances, different temperatures and the presence of tiny air bubbles in suspension have all been suggested. This contrast effect disappears when the "medium" reaches the pulmonary and peripheral capillary beds.

The contrast substance is injected as an embolus in a peripheral vein. In the absence of a right-to-left intracardiac shunt, only the right heart cavities are opacified. The visualisation of the left heart cavities is diagnostic of a shunt and its level may also be determined (see § congenital heart disease).

1.4. THE ECHOCARDIOGRAPHIC LABORATORY

Ideally, the echocardiography laboratory should dispose of one room for examination of patients and another for interpretation and filing of records; and it should be located as near to the intensive care unit and other wards as possible.

1.4.1. Choice of echocardiograph

This is fundamental. The first step is to define the service needs: routine studies, research projects, versitility (recording of other trackings such as the phonocardiogram), mobility, the need for two-dimensional echo and, above all, taking into account the necessity of a rapid and efficient after-sales service.

• **M mode**

Commercially available echocardiographs are nowadays generally of good quality: a variable speed fiber optic strip chart recorder, a large M mode screen with a degree of storage and an A mode screen for the setting of depth scale and gain control are essential. Care should be taken to choose an M mode system compatible with a two-dimensional system, if this is to be added at a later date.

None of the currently available systems is ideal. Mechanical sector scans have good proximal resolution, are more mobile and less costly than electronic systems; however, with phased array, simultaneous M mode becomes possible, the transducer may be easier to use and dynamic focussing may be available.

This comparison has been simplified as, in fact, the characteristics of each system may differ significantly from make to make. The recording is made on magnetic tape, and so the choice of recorder is critical: this may be influenced by the presence of a preexisting video system. The quality of image is related to the band width 3/4 inch gives better image restitution than 1/2 inch tape.

A photographic system is a useful accessory, polaroid being the method offered by most manufacturers. More advanced equipment is necessary for better quality reproductions; for example, digital scan converters to freeze the image.

Finally, it is essential to try out as many echocardiographs as possible. The machine offering the best value for money, taking the service needs into consideration, will then be chosen.

1.4.2. Organisation of the laboratory

A set of transducers, each with a different frequency and focal length, is useful for M mode echocardiography. Transducers of 2,25 MHz frequency and focal length of 7,5 cm, are generally used to examine adults, whereas frequencies of 3,5 and 5 MHz are more appropriate for the examination of children and babies. These characteristics should be checked annually by the manufacturer.

Technicians may be employed to help position the patient and even to record the echocardiogram, under medical supervision, when a high patient turnover is expected. The echocardiogram may be reported on a standard printed sheet showing the normal values for the laboratory.

Three examinations a day is the minimum level of activity (American Heart Association[164]) to maintain the quality of a laboratory's results.

With the growth of the computer industry, systems of automatic analysis have become available[209]. These programs provide detailed analysis of left ventricular function (for research projects), but some systems may also be used for an automatic printout of results, and for administrative purposes.

1.4.3. Limitations of echocardiography

As previously mentioned, ultrasound is absorbed by air and bone. Echocardiography is often difficult in obese and emphysematous patients, and in those with deformities of the chest wall. However, by multiplying the number of incidences of M mode and two-dimensional examination, interpretable recordings may be obtained from almost all patients.

Even when the recording is of poor quality, some simple problems may be resolved in most cases. The experience, skill and application of the operator play an important role.

CHAPTER 2
ECHOCARDIOGRAPHIC EXAMINATION

2.1. ECHOCARDIOGRAPHIC ANATOMY

The heart may be imagined situated within the thoracic cavity with an oblique long axis running from its apex to its base[54]. This axis, therefore, passes through the left ventricle and outflow tract and is partially surrounded by the right ventricle. Its obliquity changes from patient to patient. This long axis forms the echocardiographic landmark for the rest of the examination, the left heart cavities being scanned from the apex of the left ventricle to the aorta, and the other structures being studied in transverse views at various levels perpendicular to the long axis[200].

In order to avoid interference due to lung intersecting the ultrasonic beam, the transducer has to be positioned over "acoustic windows", usually located in an intercostal space in the left parasternal region, at the apex and subcostal area (Plate I).

2.2. POSITIONING THE PATIENT

The patient is placed on a bed of convenient height for the operator to be able to examine him or her comfortably. An ECG is connected. The examination is started in the supine position, but the patient may have to be turned into his left side, which brings the heart closer to the chest wall, in order to record good quality M mode tracings and to facilitate the location of the apex for apical views. The examination is easier with the operator on the patient's left side, holding the transducer in his left hand and adjusting the echocardiographic controls with his right hand. The different oscilloscopes are best viewed under dimmed light.

A water soluble ultrasonic gel is used to obtain an airless contact between the transducer and the skin.

2.3. RECORDING TECHNIQUE

The «acoustic window», especially for M mode recordings, is usually located in the third or fourth left intercostal space; this is where the investigation is started. The examination should be completed with routine apical and subcostal recordings[200].

2.3.1. Parasternal views

A) *Long axis* (plate II)

This view allows the study of the aorta, mitral valve, left ventricle and left atrium[54].

These structures may be recorded by M mode scanning. The transducer is placed perpendicular to the chest wall to visualise the mitral valve, and then gradually angled towards the right shoulder to bring the aorta into view, and towards the apex to record the left ventricle.

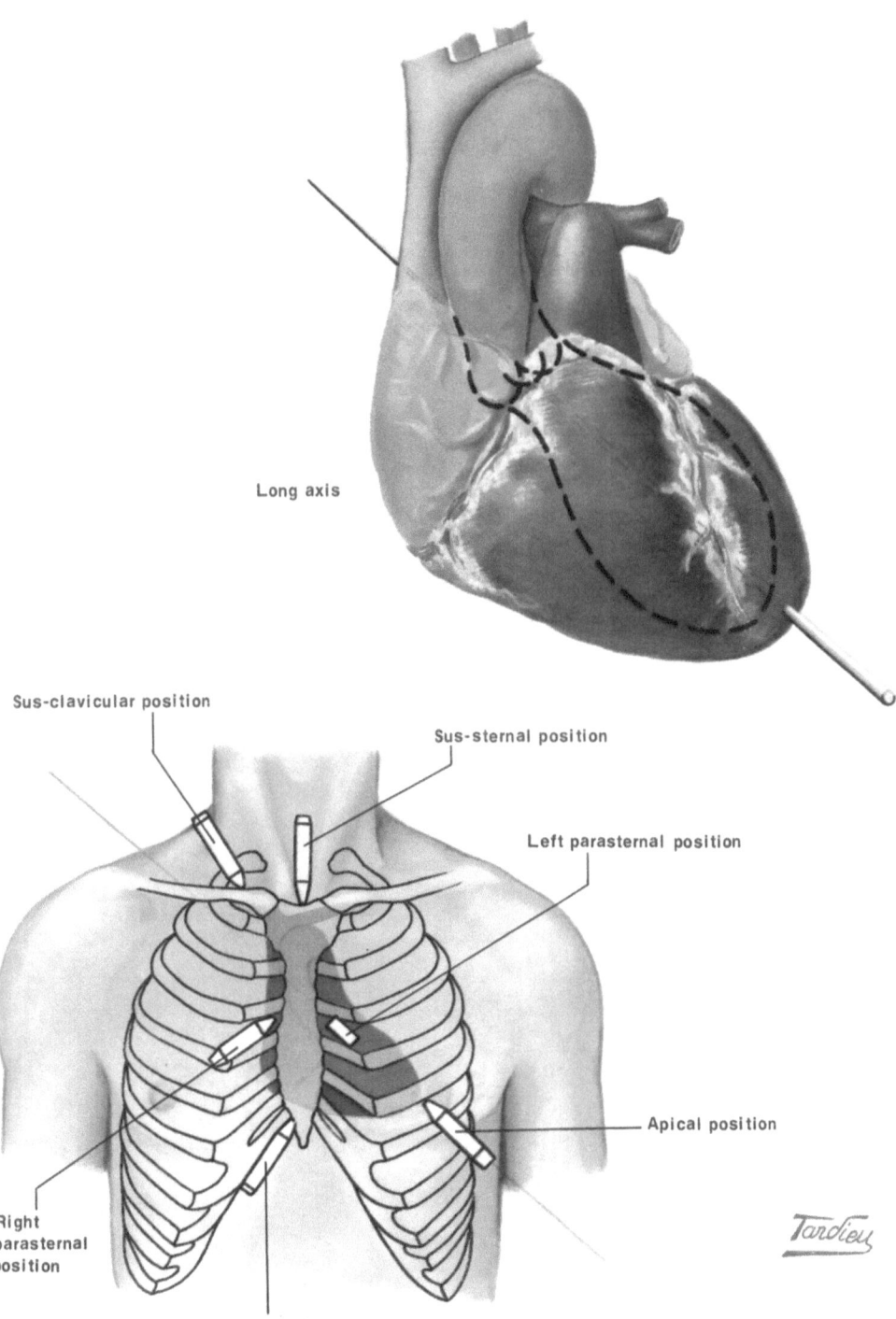

Long axis

Sus-clavicular position

Sus-sternal position

Left parasternal position

Apical position

Right parasternal position

Sub-costal position

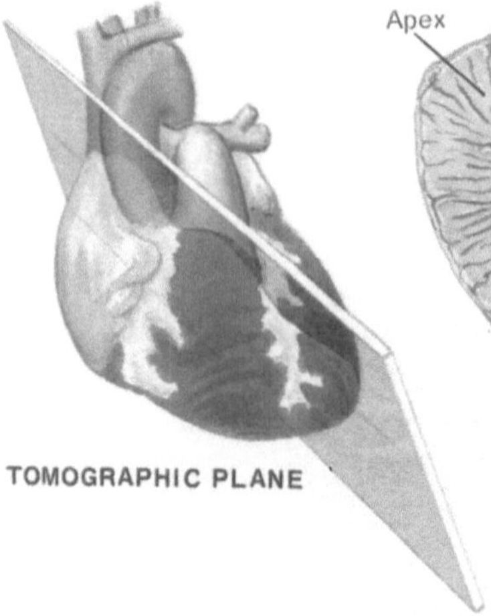

TOMOGRAPHIC PLANE

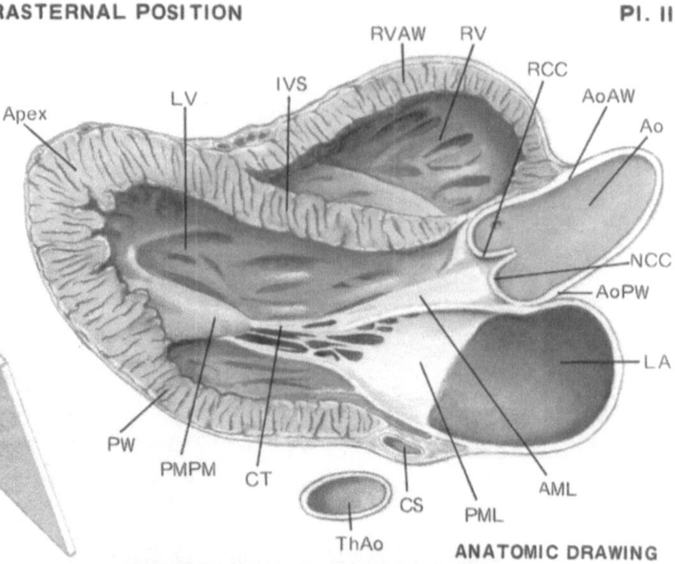

Apex · LV · IVS · RVAW · RV · RCC · AoAW · Ao · NCC · AoPW · LA · AML · PML · CS · ThAo · CT · PMPM · PW

ANATOMIC DRAWING

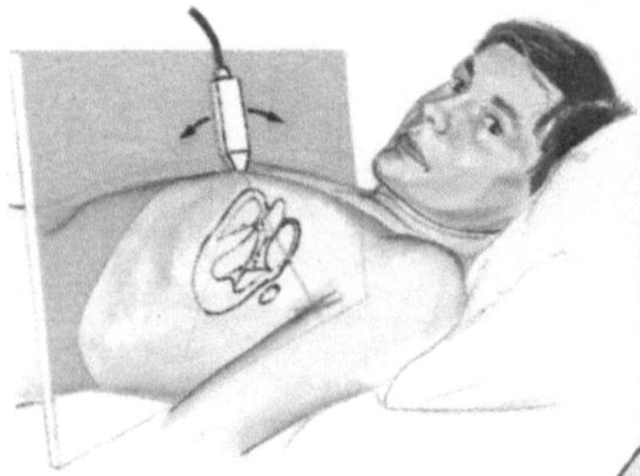

POSITION AND ORIENTATION OF THE TRANSDUCER

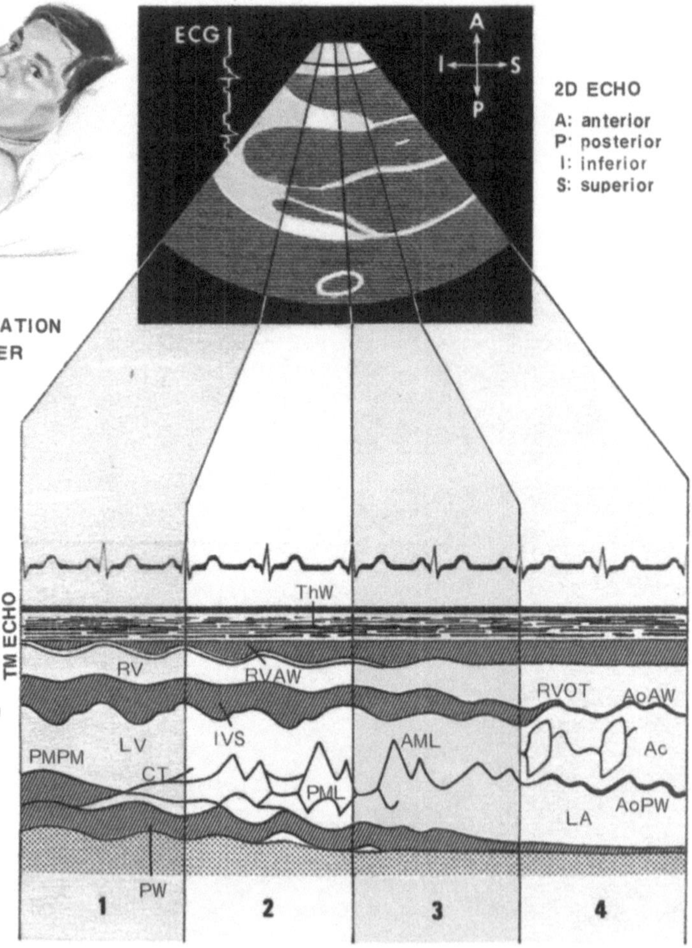

ECG

2D ECHO

A: anterior
P: posterior
I: inferior
S: superior

Ao   = aorta
AoAW = aortic anterior wall
AoPW = aortic posterior wall
ThAo = thoracic aorta
RCC   = right coronary cusp
NCC   = non coronary cusp
AML   = anterior mitral leaflet
PML   = posterior mitral leaflet
CT   = chordae tendinae
LA   = left atrium
PW   = posterior wall
PMPM = postero-medial
        papillary muscle
IVS   = interventricular septum
RV   = right ventricle
RVAN = right ventricle
        anterior wall
LV   = left ventricle
ThW   = thoracic wall
CS   = coronary sinus
RVOT = right ventricular
        outflow tract

TM ECHO

ThW · RV · RVAW · RVOT · AoAW · PMPM · LV · IVS · AML · Ac · CT · PML · LA · AoPW · PW

1   2   3   4

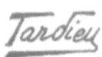

B) *Short axis* (plate III, IV, V)

The views are perpendicular (the transducer is rotated through 90°) to the long axis. They are recorded at different levels from the base to the apex of the heart by gradually changing the angle of the sector scan.

- position 1, the transverse view passes through the papillary muscles;

- position 2, the beam passes through the short transverse axis of the left ventricle at the free edge of mitral valve leaflets;

- position 3, the mitral annulus comes into view;

- position 4, the great vessels are recorded anteriorly and the atria, posteriously.

In M mode, the tricuspid valve may be recorded from position 4 by tilting the transducer caudally, and the pulmonary valve, by tilting towards the left shoulder, the aorta being approximately situated halfway between the two (plate V).

2.3.2. Apical views

These views are mainly confined to two-dimensional echocardiography as they are very difficult to interpret in M mode.

They are as important as the parasternal views as all four chambers and the two atrioventricular valves may be visualised simultaneously[177]. The aorta may also be recorded.

With the patient in the left lateral position, the transducer is placed over the apex beat, and the examining plane directed upwards, towards the right shoulder. This is, in fact, another long axis view from the apex to the base of the heart. Two perpendicular planes may be defined[177] [200], one taking in the four chambers (plate VI) and the other, at 90°, taking in the left atrium and ventricle, a view which is the echocardiographic equivallence of the right anterior oblique angiographic incidence of the left heart cavities (plate VII).

Apical views are essential for the assessment of left ventricular performance. They are easier to record in patients with easily palpable apex beats irrespective of the shape of the chest wall.

In M mode, they are mainly used to determine the maximum amplitude of prosthetic heart valves motion.

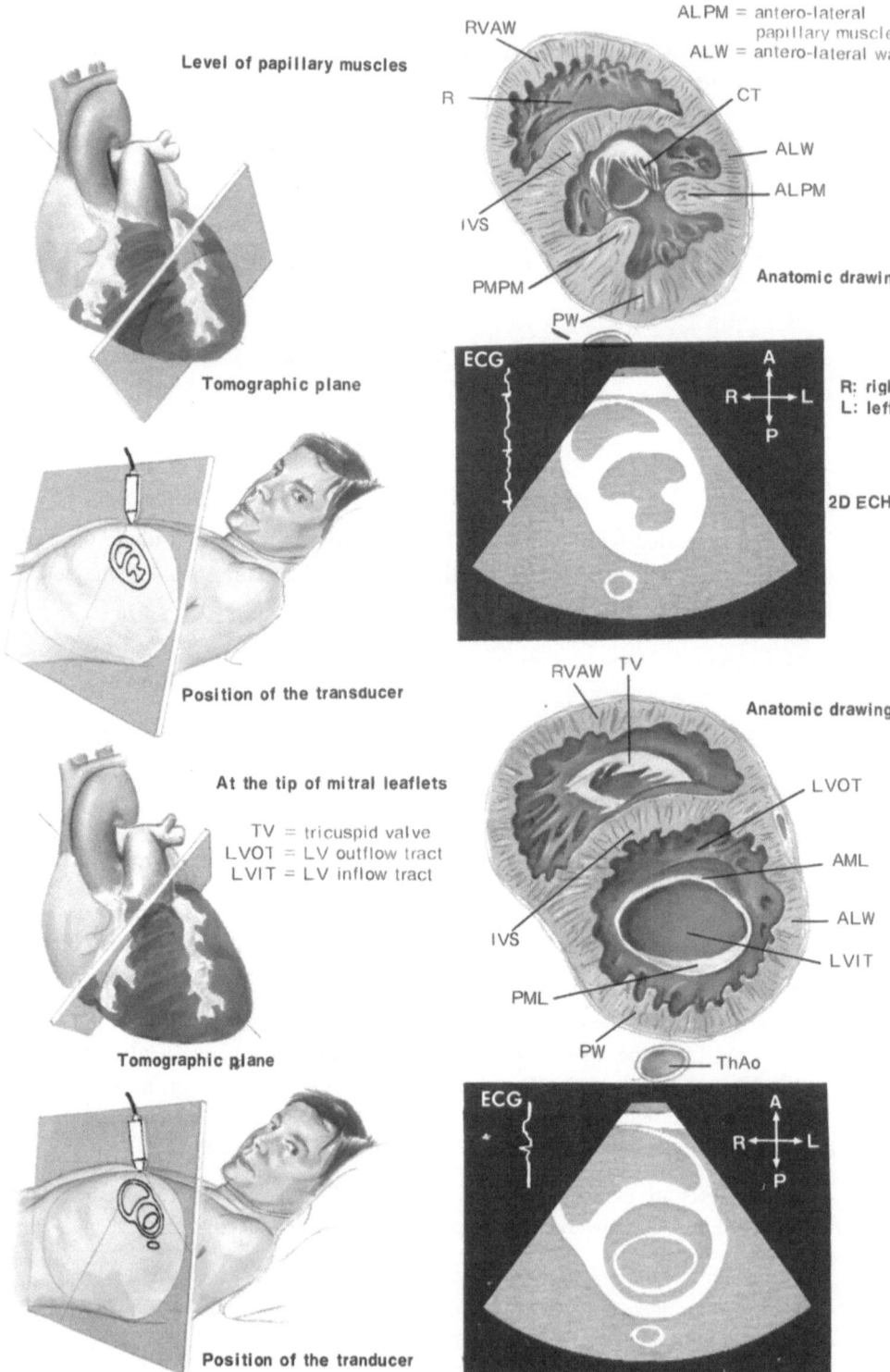

AL.PM = antero-lateral papillary muscle
ALW = antero-lateral wall

Level of papillary muscles

RVAW

R

CT

ALW

AL.PM

IVS

PMPM

PW

Anatomic drawing

Tomographic plane

ECG

A

R ←→ L

P

R: right
L: left

2D ECHO

Position of the transducer

At the tip of mitral leaflets

TV = tricuspid valve
LVOT = LV outflow tract
LVIT = LV inflow tract

RVAW   TV

Anatomic drawing

LVOT

AML

ALW

LVIT

IVS

PML

PW

ThAo

Tomographic plane

ECG

A

R ←→ L

P

Position of the tranducer

Tardieu

Anatomic drawing

At the level of
the LV outflow tract

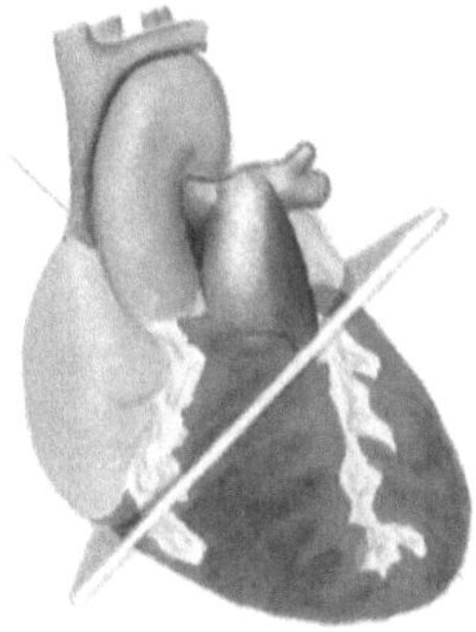

Tomographic plane

RA = right atrium

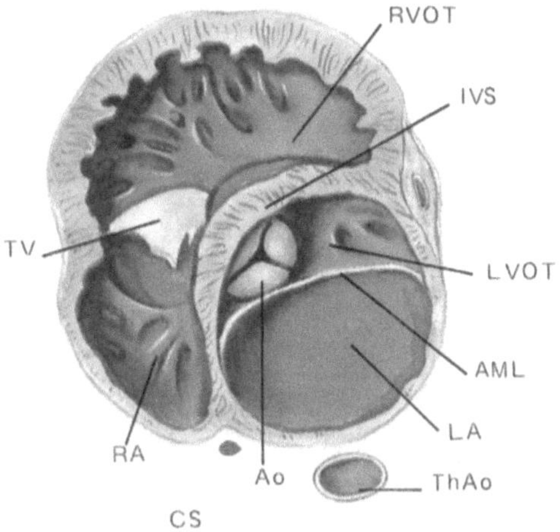

RVOT

IVS

TV

LVOT

AML

LA

RA

Ao   ThAo

CS

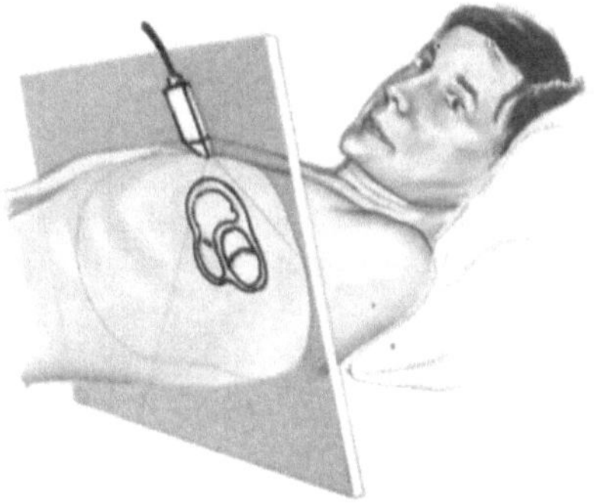

Position of the transducer

ECG

A

R ←→ L

P

2D ECHO

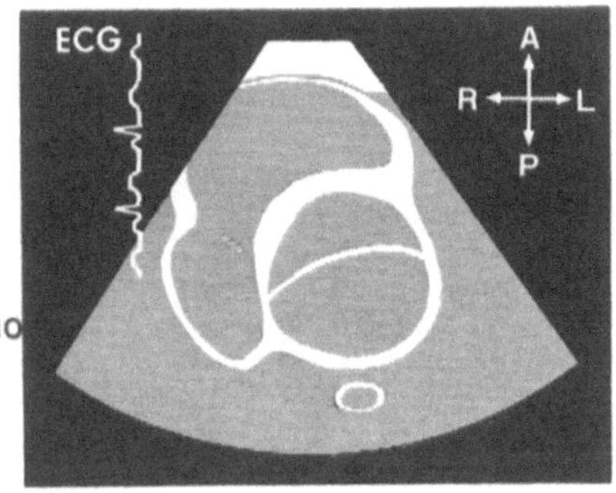

Tardieu

At the base

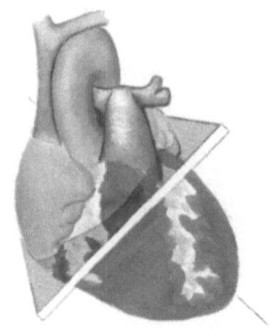

Tomagraphic plane

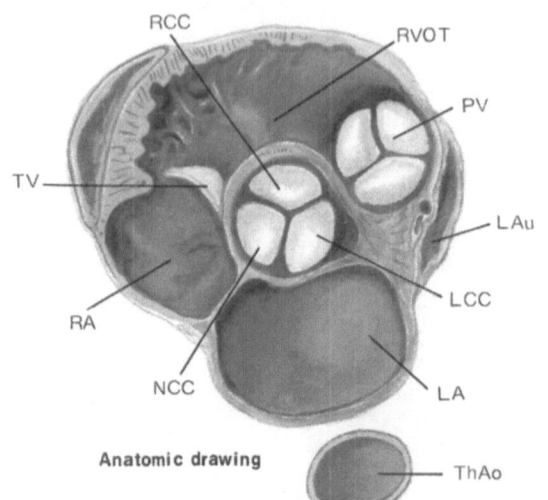

Anatomic drawing

Position of the transducer

ECG

2D ECHO

LCC = left coronary cusp
PV = pulmonary valve
RA = right atrium
LAu = left auricle

Tardieu

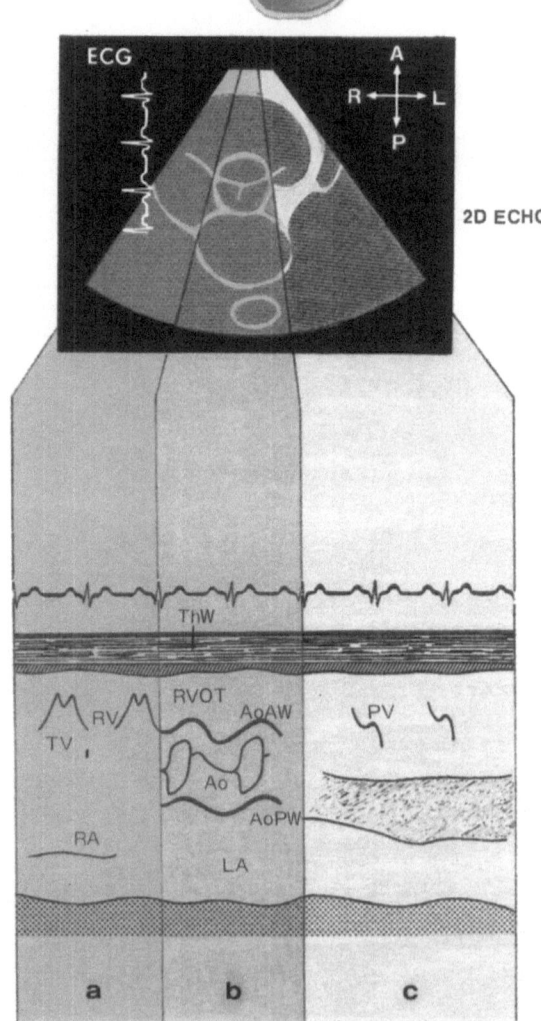

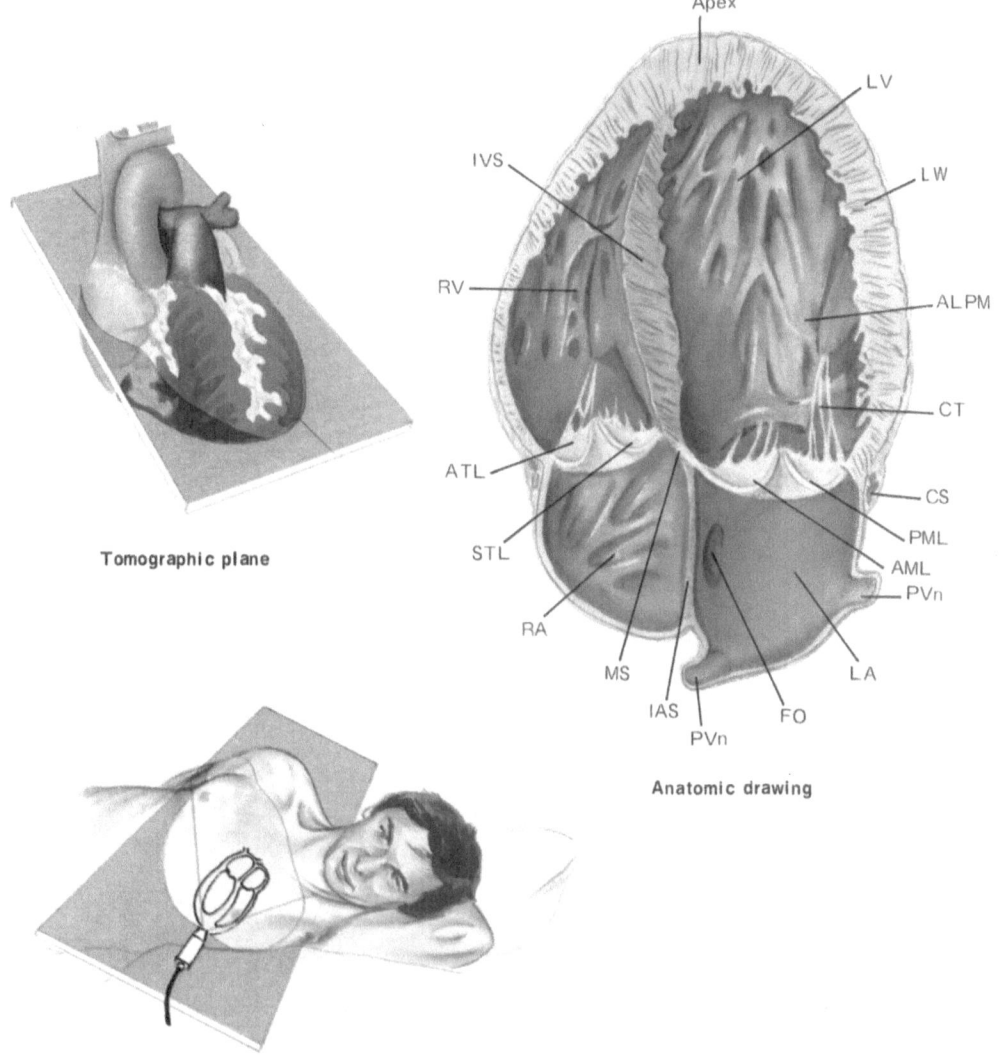

Tomographic plane

Anatomic drawing

Apex · LV · IVS · LW · RV · AL PM · CT · ATL · CS · STL · PML · AML · RA · PVn · MS · LA · IAS · FO · PVn

Position of the transducer

ATL = anterior tricuspid leaflet
STL = septal tricuspid leaflet
FO = fossa ovalis
IAS = inter atrial septum
PVn = pulmonary vein
MS = membranous septum

2D ECHO

ECG

Apex
R ←→ L
Base

Tardieu

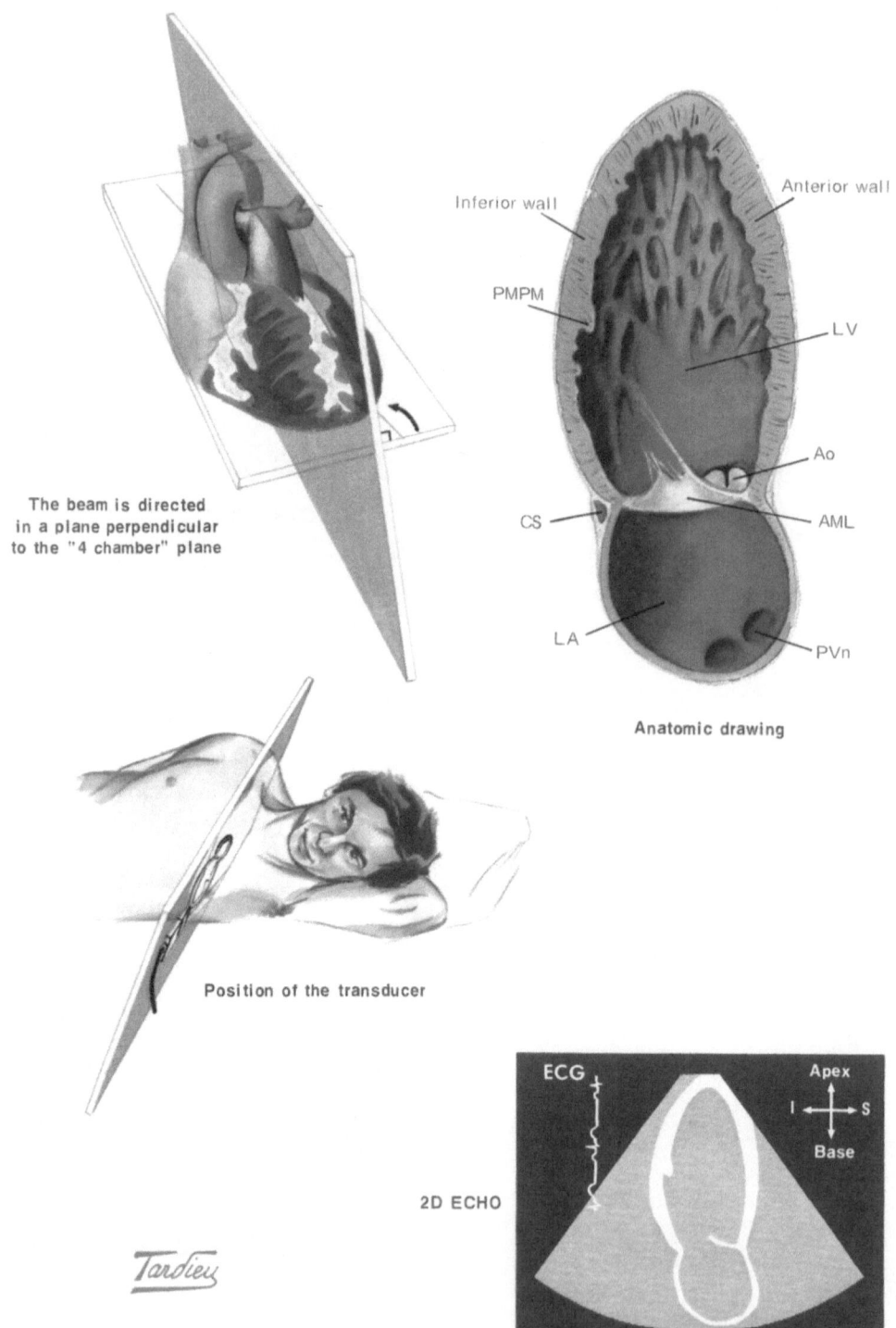

The beam is directed
in a plane perpendicular
to the "4 chamber" plane

Inferior wall

Anterior wall

PMPM

LV

CS

Ao

AML

LA

PVn

Anatomic drawing

Position of the transducer

2D ECHO

ECG

Apex

I ←→ S

Base

Tardieu

2.3.3. Subcostal views

The patient is placed on his back with his legs fexed to relax the abdominal muscles (deep inspiration is sometimes useful), and the transducer placed in the subcostal area. Scanning through a horizontal plane visualises the heart along its long axis (plate VIII), and the four cardiac chambers may be recorded[200]. Rotation through 90° gives the various transverse views (plate IX), extending as far as the right atrium and the inferior veina cava[124]. Increased angulation of the transducer towards the right side is required (see fig. 3-34).

This position is also used for M mode and is very useful when the parasternal views are unobtainable[24].

A long axis view, morphologically comparable to the usual M mode scan, may be recorded; but it must be appreciated that other myocardial zones are being visualised (inferior portion of the interventricular septum, and lateral wall of the left ventricle).

The motion of the interatrial septum may be also recorded by two-dimensional imaging with simultaneous M mode tracings.

2.3.4. Accessory views (plate I)

Other echocardiographic views may be obtained by positioning the transducer in the suprasternal notch, to visualise the aortic arch, right pulmonary artery and the left atrium[71 72]; the right supra-clavicular fossa, for analysis of the amplitude of aortic valve prostheses motion [25 238]; the right parasternal area, for the recording of the interatrial septum[149 201]; and the left precordial area for the M mode study of the left ventricular anterior wall[33].

2.4. PRESENTATION OF 2D RECORDINGS: RECOMMENDATIONS OF THE AMERICAN SOCIETY OF ECHOCARDIOGRAPHY (*Circulation*, **62**:212, 1980).

The American Society of Echocardiography recommends the following presentation :

Long-axis views

The patient is seen from the left side with the head (and therefore the ascending aorta) to the right (plate II).

Short-axis views

The heart is seen from the apex, the right ventricle being to the left and the left ventricle to the right of the recording (plate III, IV, V).

Apical views

The same presentation as for the short axis views is used for the 4-chamber view (plate VI). For the RAO equivalent, a presentation similar to that for the long axis views is recommended. (plate VII)

The other views, suprasternal and subcostal, are presented according to the same principle (plate VIII, IX).

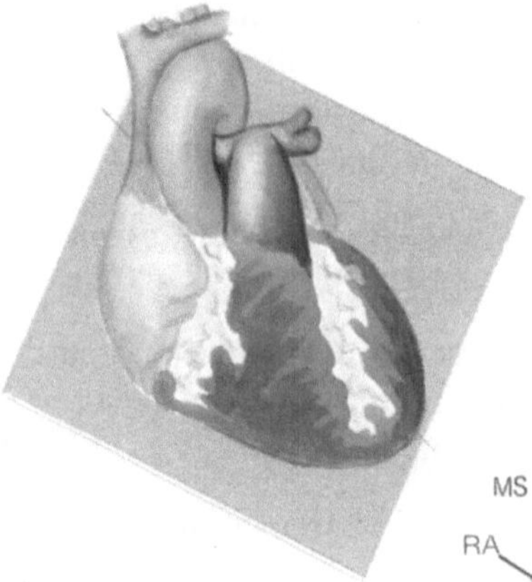

Tomographic plane

Anatomic drawing

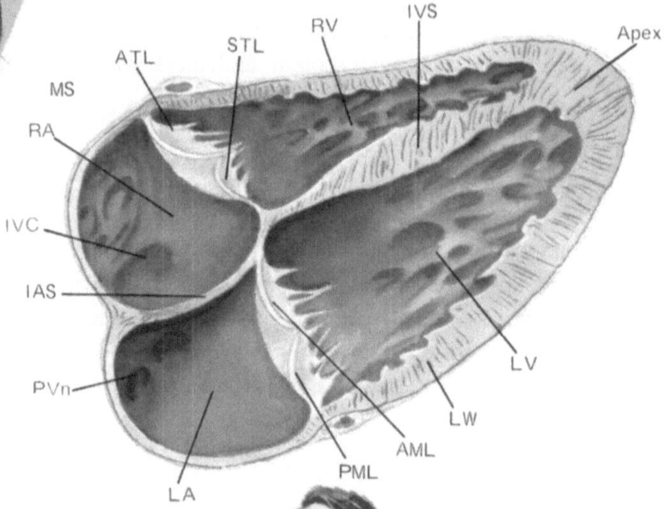

RV
IVS
Apex
ATL
STL
MS
RA
IVC
IAS
PVn
LA
PML
AML
LW
LV

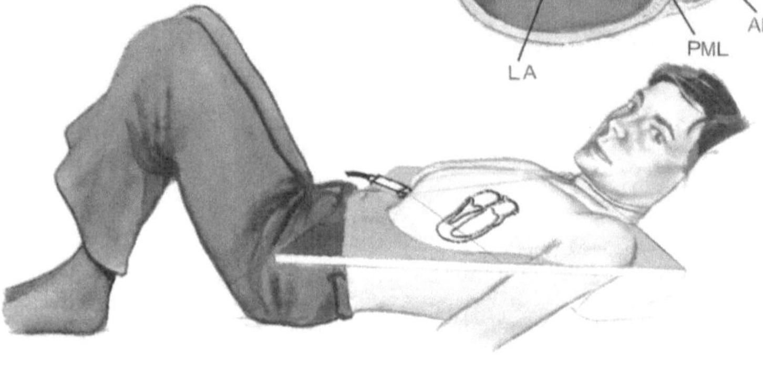

Position of the transducer

IVC = Inferior vena cava

2D ECHO

ECG
I
Apex
Liver
Base
S

Tardieu

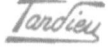

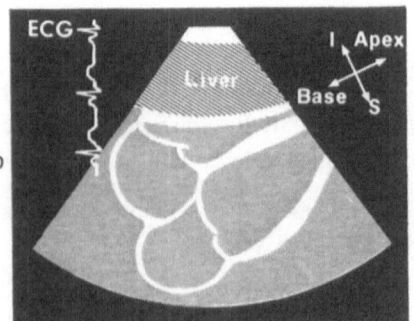

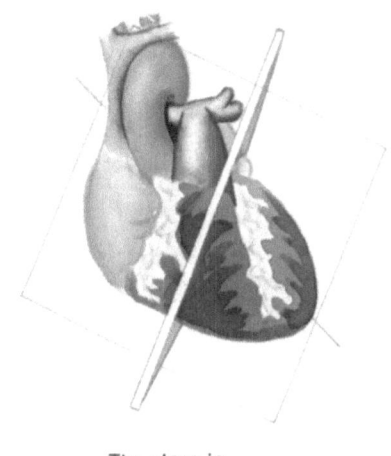

The plane is
perpendicular to the sub-costal
"4 chamber" plane

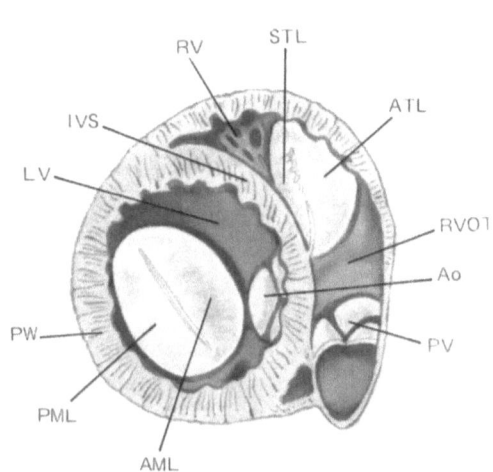

Anatomic drawing

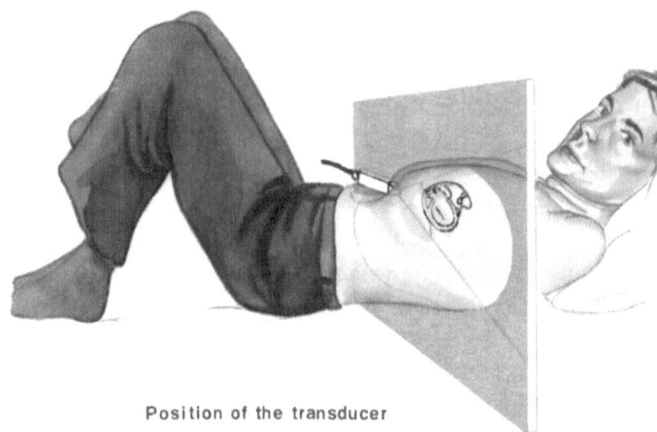

Position of the transducer

2D ECHO

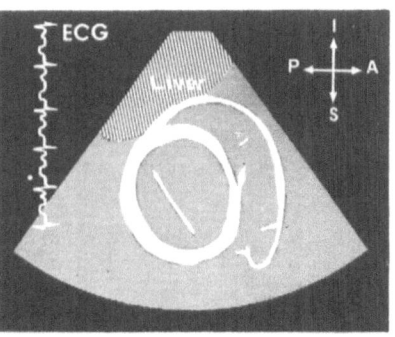

CHAPTER 3

THE NORMAL ECHOCARDIOGRAM

3.1. THE HEART VALVES

3.1.1. Mitral Valve

The echos of the mitral valve are a useful landmark for the rest of the echocardiographic examination. They usually are the easiest to record and, from a historical point of view, they were among the first to be described[48].

A) *2D long axis view* (Plate II)

The whole of the mitral mitral apparatus from the papillary muscles to the left atrium may be visualised. Long axis views may be recorded from the three routine transducer positions, but the best images are generally obtained with the transducer in the left parasternal region.

Valvular motion is difficult to study from still frames. The extreme positions of the mitral leaflets in systole and diastole and their precise motion on M mode recording will be analysed. This method will also be used for the other heart valves.

- **Diastole**

This is the period of left ventricular filling : the mitral valve is open and the aortic valve closed (fig. 3-1).

In early diastole, the anterior mitral leaflet has a rapid anterior motion towards the interventricular septum. The posterior leaflet moves in the opposite direction but with less amplitude. The mitral ring also has a slight posterior motion. During this phase, the maximum separation of the two valves usually attains about 30 mm. The echos of the anterior leaflet are in continuity with the posterior wall of the aorta wich, from the echocardiographic point of view, forms the anterior wall of the left atrium; the posterior leaflet is in echocardiographic continuity with the posterior wall of the left atrium. As they open, the two leaflets move down into the left ventricular cavity, defining the left ventricular inflow tract between the two leaflets, and the outflow tract above the anterior mitral leaflet.

- **Systole**

At the onset of ventricular contraction, the mitral valve closes and the two leaflets come together (fig. 3-2).

The angle[70] between the axis of the aortic posterior wall and the anterior mitral leaflet should not exceed 30°. The mitral ring has a slight anterior motion. The echocardiographic continuity of the posterior leaflet with the chordae and the posterior median papillary muscle is often well visualised (tilting the transducer medially helps bring them into view). The distance between the free edge of the mitral valve and the papillary muscle may therefore be measured in systole.

The thickness of the valves and chordae may also be assessed.

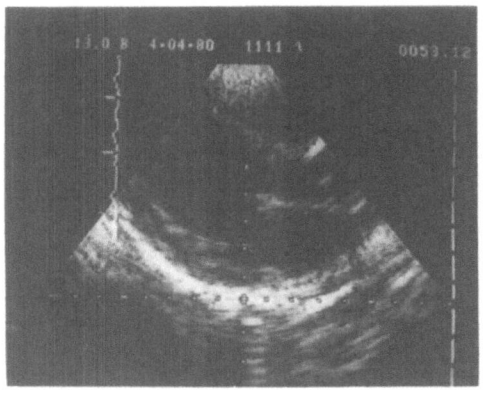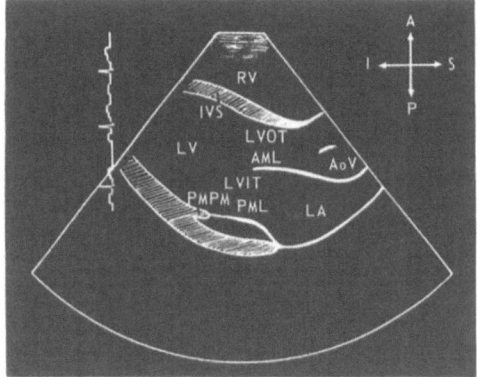

Fig. 3-1 2D long axis view of the mitral valve in diastole
LVOT: left ventricle outflow tract
LVIT : left ventricle inflow tract
PMPM: postero-medial papillary muscle

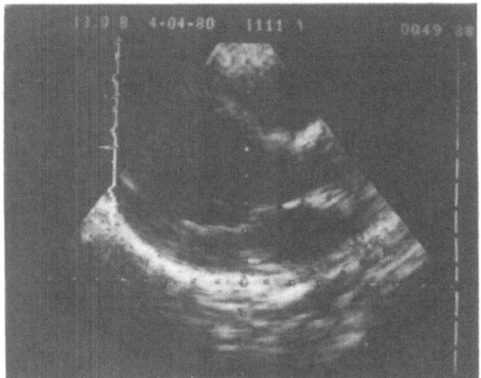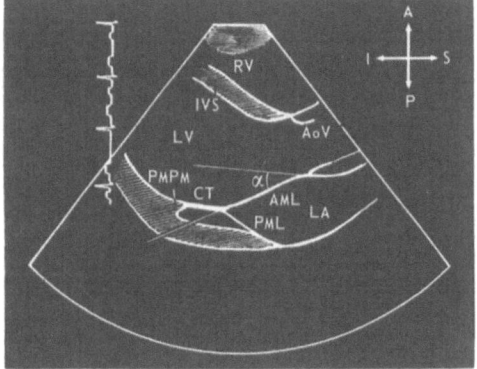

Fig. 3-2 2D long axis view of the mitral valve in systole
CT: chordae tendinae

Approximately the same appearances are obtained by recording from the subcostal area; the apical view, however, visualises these structures from one of the extremities of the long axis.

B) *2D short axis* (fig. 3-3, 3-4, plate III).

This view is recorded from the left parasternal area, in a plane perpendicular to the long axis (alternatively, the subcostal position may be used). Its principal advantage is that a good view of the mitral orifice is obtained in diastole, as the plane passes through the free border of the mitral leaflets[89] [133]. The orifice is oval in shape and has been likened to a fish's mouth; the surface area of the valve may be obtained by planimetry. It should be performed on a view in early diastole, when the mitral leaflets are furthest apart, and care must be taken to adjust the gain control so that the leaflets do not appear artefactually thickened[133]. The anterolateral and posterior commissures form the two extremities of this ellipsoid.

37

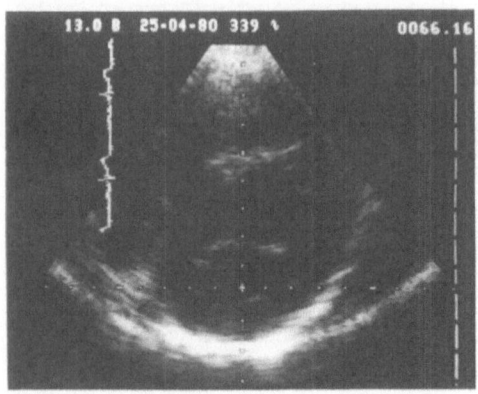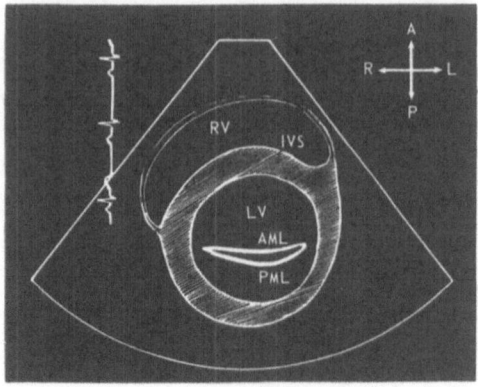

Fig. 3-3 2D short axis view of the mitral valve in diastole

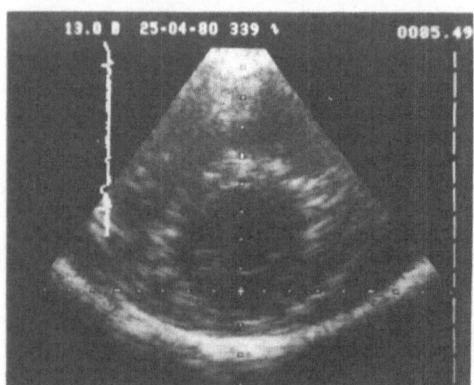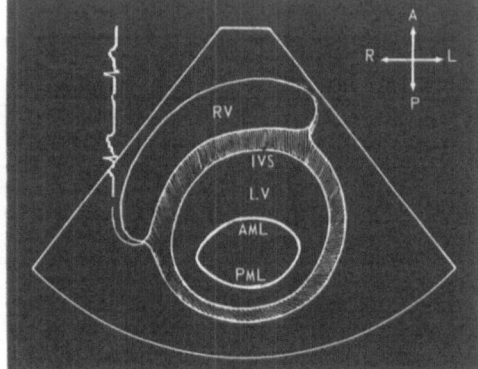

Fig. 3-4 2D short axis view of the mitral valve in systole

In systole, the closure of the mitral valve with apposition of the two leaflets all along the width of the mitral orifice, should be verified. The same echocardiographic continuity is observed on mitro-aortic scanning.

C) M Mode

The M-shaped appearance of the anterior mitral leaflet in diastole is a very characteristic echocardiographic feature.

The successive phases of this echo have been described and defined by previous workers[48] [54] [130]:

— The DE phase: the anterior leaflet has a rapid anterior motion as far as its point of maximal excursion, the E point. The leaflet may sometimes touch the left border of the interventricular septum at this point. It then starts to close, the end point of early diastolic closure being known as the F point. When diastole is long, the leaflet remains in a partially open position until atrial contraction leads to reopening of the leaflet as far as the A point. In general, the amplitude of presystolic opening is smaller than that of the early diastolic

Fig. 3-5

Normal mitral valve echogram
RVW: right ventricle wall

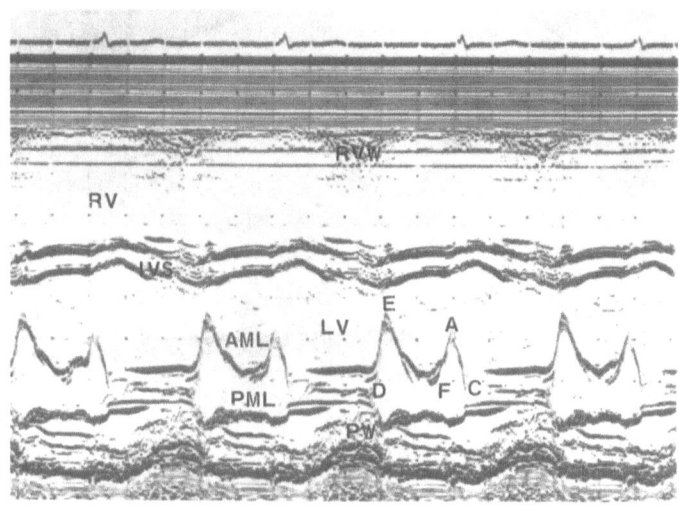

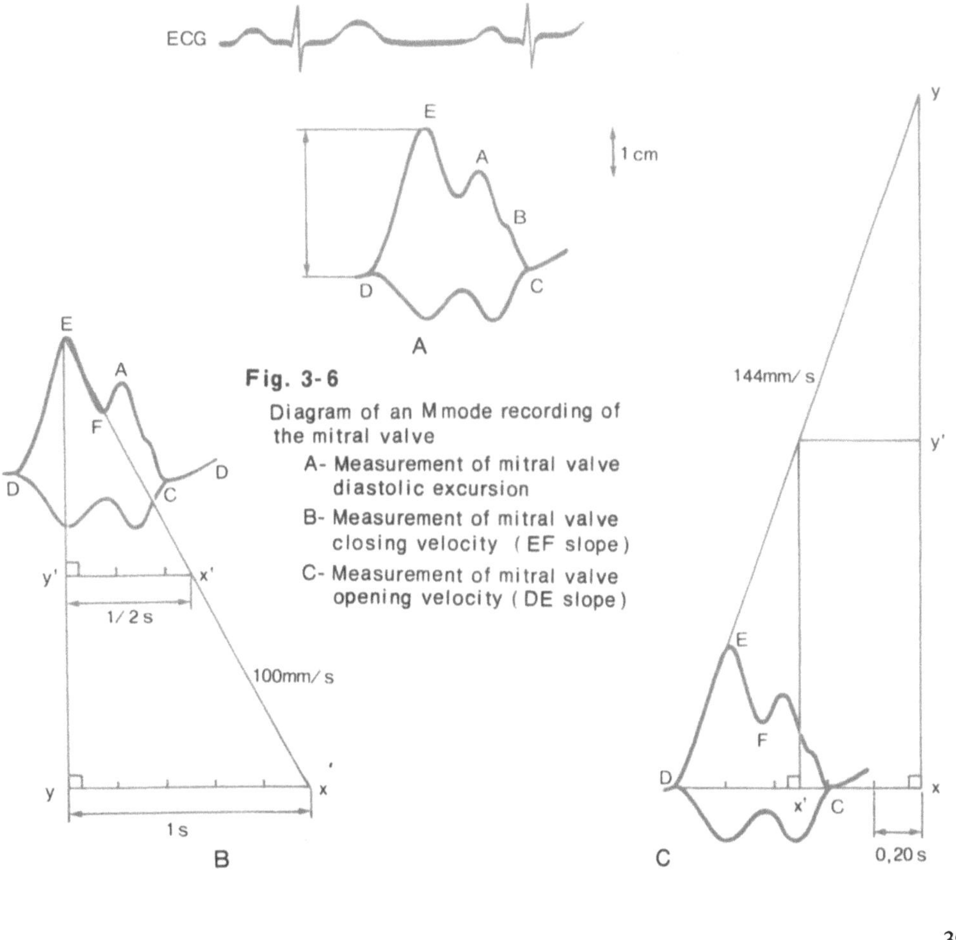

Fig. 3-6

Diagram of an M mode recording of the mitral valve

A- Measurement of mitral valve diastolic excursion

B- Measurement of mitral valve closing velocity (EF slope)

C- Measurement of mitral valve opening velocity (DE slope)

opening. The leaflet then tends to close before the onset of ventricular systole. A "B" point may be observed in certain pathological conditions before the leaflet finally closes at the C point. During systole, the anterior leaflet has a slight anterior motion from the C to the D point due to the overall anterior displacement of the left ventricle[155] [159] [169] [205] (fig. 3-5).

The posterior leaflet is smaller and more difficult to record. During diastole, it has a posterior "mirror image" motion with respect to the anterior leaflet, but of smaller amplitude. During systole, it rejoins the anterior leaflet, and the two leaflets remain together throughout the CD phase[23].

The appearances of the mitral echos depend on the position of the transducer: M mode scanning from the left ventricle to the aorta also shows their continuity with the other cardiac structures. The maximum excursion of the leaflets is observed at the junction of the left ventricle and atrium[218]. Their amplitude decreases as scanning is continued towards the aorta, the anterior leaflet being in continuity with the posterior aortic wall. Similarly, the echos of the posterior mitral leaflet disappear as the beam is scanned from the papillary muscles to the aorta (fig 3-7, fig 3-29).

Therefore, the correct incidence for analysis of mitral valve echos is when both leaflets are recorded just before the posterior leaflet echos disappear.

Various measurements of the mitral valve echos may be made: fig. 3-6 shows how the EF slope is measured. Its values reflects the haemodynamic conditions during the passive phase of left ventricular filling and the normal range is from 80 to 150 mm/sec.[36] [98] [113] [121]. The amplitude of excursion of the mitral valve is measured from the D to the E point (fig. 3-6): the normal values ranges between 20 and 30 mm.

Different echos of the mitral valve are often recorded simultaneously; this superposition sometimes gives rise to echos which are difficult to interpret. Echos recorded from above or below the leaflets: e.g. anterior or posterior chordae, part of the mitral annulus or even one structure recorded several times, are examples of the problem of lateral resolution of the ultrasound beam[165].

3.1.2. Aorta and Aortic Valve

The aortic root and aortic cusps are normally recorded in routine examinations.

A) *2D long axis view* (fig. 3-9, 3-10, plate II)

This view is obtained with the transducer positioned in the left parasternal area; the proximal aorta and the sinus of Valsalva, the anterior and posterior aortic walls with their parallel motion, and the 2 to 3 cm above the aortic valve may be recorded. During systole, these structures have an anterior motion[177].

Two of the aortic cusps are visualised in this plane (the right coronary and the posterior or non-coronary cusp)[54]. During diastole (fig. 3-9), the valves are closed giving rise to a single echo equidistant from the two walls of the aorta. In systole (fig. 3-10), the valve opens and the echos of the two cusps separate, the anterior cusp moving anteriorly to the anterior wall and the posterior cusp moving posteriorly to the posterior wall, each leaving a slight gap

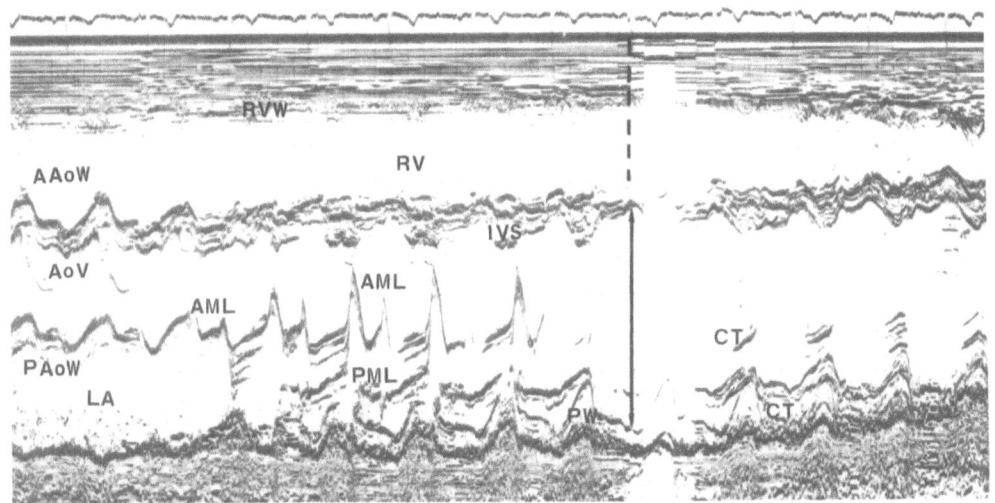

Fig. 3-7 Mmode scan showing normal continuity between the aortic posterior
wall and the anterior mitral leaflet
AAoW: anterior aortic wall
PAoW: posterior aortic wall

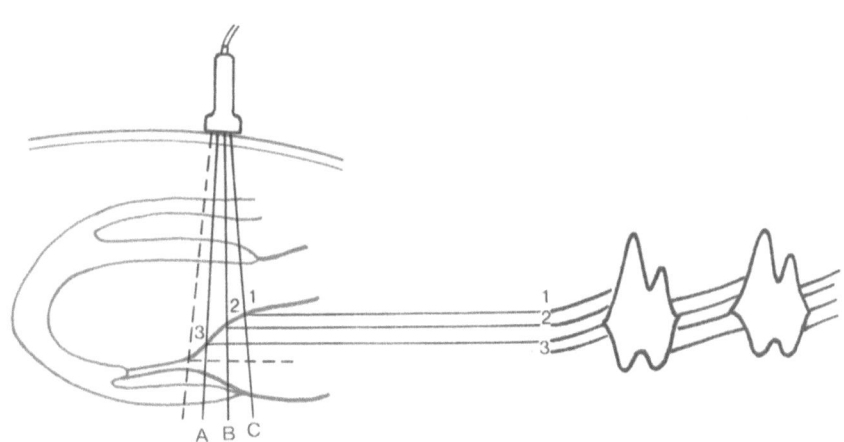

Fig. 3-8 Mmode recording of the mitral valve illustrating the problem of lateral resolution.
Divergence of the ultrasonic beam is responsible for the recording of multiple
echos from three points on the anterior mitral leaflet.

corresponding to the sinus of Valsalva The continuity of the anterior wall of the aorta and the
interventricular septum, and of the posterior wall of the aorta and the anterior mitral leaflet, is
particularly well seen in long axis views[200].

41

The descending thoracic aorta is visualised as an oval echo-free space behind the heart plate II, Fig. 3-9 and 3-10). It may be followed down to the abdominal aorta by angling the transducer in the sagittal plane; this manœuvre differentiates it from other causes of a retrocardiac echo-free space (fig. 3-11).

It is possible, especially in children, to record the origin of the aorta and the aortic arch from the subcostal position by orientating the transducer obliquely upwards (fig. 3-12)[11].

The aortic arch, the origin of the cerebral vessels and the right pulmonary artery may be visualised from the suprasternal notch (fig. 3-13)[200].

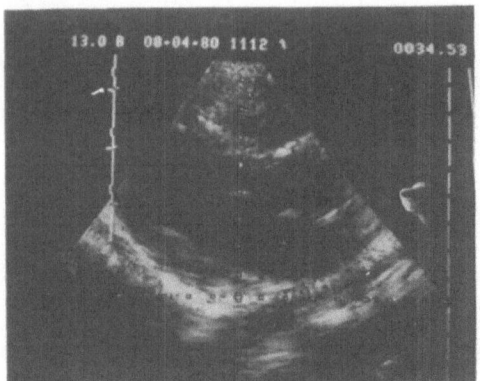 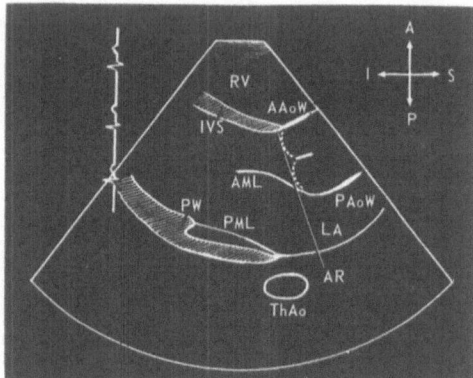

Fig. 3-9 2D long axis diastolic view of a normal aortic root
AR: aortic root
ThAo: thoracic aorta

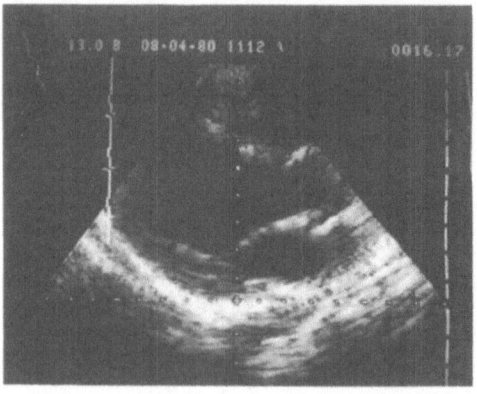 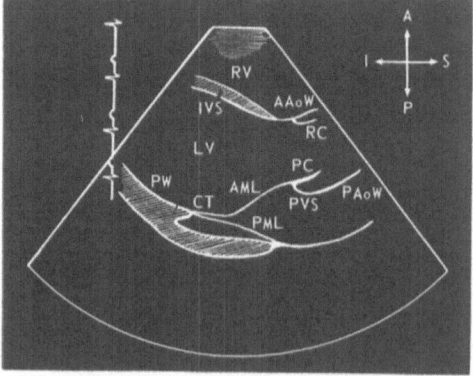

Fig. 3-10 2D long axis systolic view of a normal aortic root
RC: right cusp
PC: post. cusp
PVS: post. valsalva sinus

B) *Short axis views* (Plate V)

This view allows visualisation of all three aortic cusps: it is recorded with the transducer positioned in the left parasternal or subcostal area, with the sector plane at 90° to the long axis.

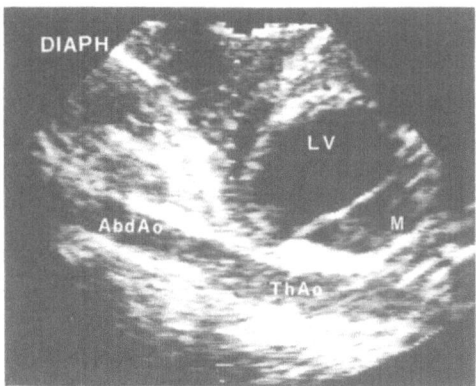

Fig. 3-11

2D parasternal sagittal view of the descending thoracic aorta (ThAo)
DIAPH: diaphragm
Abd Ao: abdominal aorta

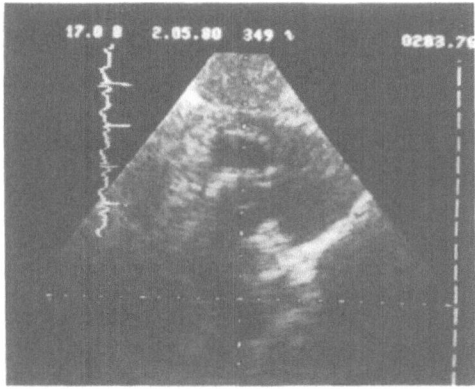 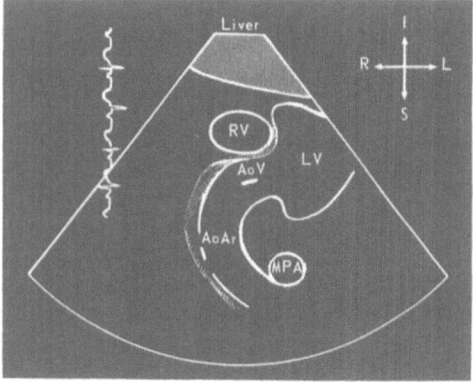

Fig. 3-12 2D subcostal view of the aortic arch
AoAr: aortic arch
MPA: main pulmonary artery

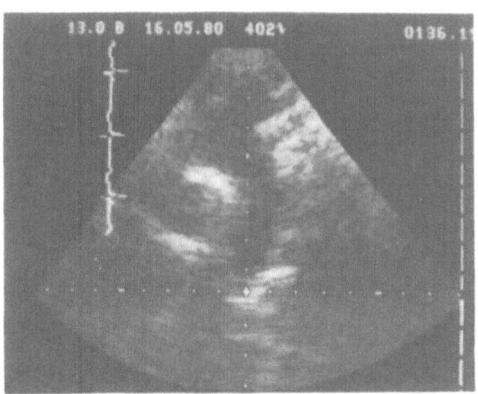 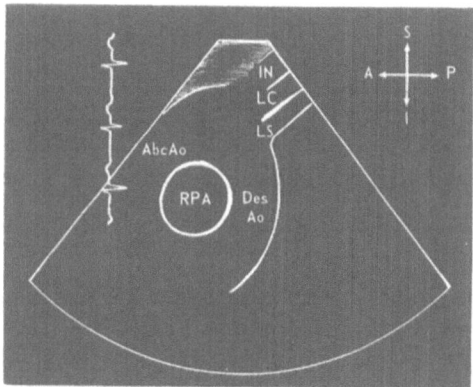

Fig. 3-13 2D suprasternal view of the aortic arch, the transducer being
orientated inferiorly and slightly posteriorly
Des Ao: descending aorta   LC: left carotid artery
Asc Ao: ascending aorta   LS: left subclavian artery
IN: innominate artery   RPA: right pulmonary artery

This gives a short axis view of the aortic ring and allows a direct assessment of its circumference (fig. 3-14).

In diastole, the aortic valve is closed and the three commissures resemble the Mercedes-Benz sign upside down[177]. They are of equal length and the central point is located at the center of the aortic ring. In systole, they separate and flatten against the aortic wall, and are difficult to visualise unless thickened by disease: the valvular surface area may be measured by planimetry.

Tilting the transducer obliquely upwards, sometimes brings the left main coronary artery into view at the center of the left coronary cusp (fig 3-15)[228]. The right coronary artery is more difficult to record as it lies anterior to the aorta. Only its ostium at the center of the right coronary cusp is visible[17].

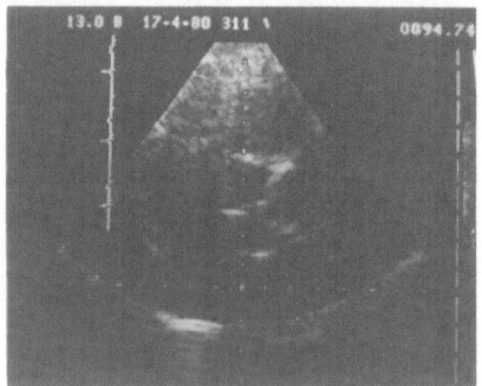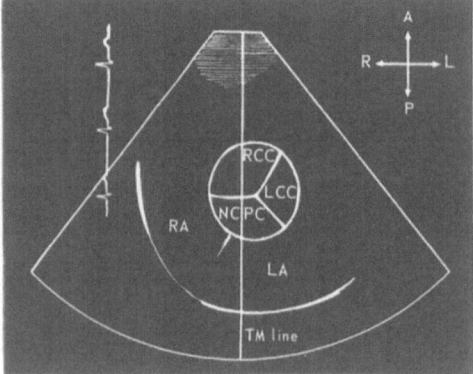

Fig. 3-14 2D parasternal short axis diastolic view of a normal aortic valve
RCC: right coronary cusp
NCPC: noncoronary post. cusp
LCC: left coronary cusp

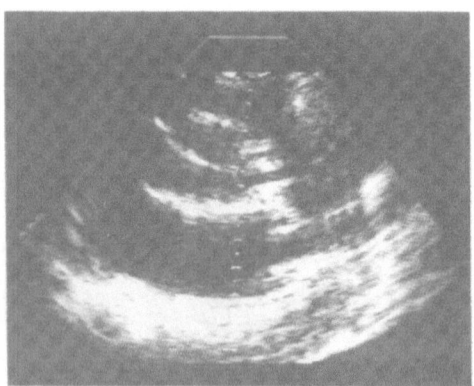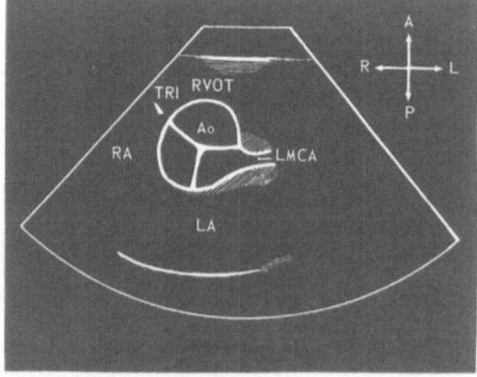

Fig. 3-15 2D short axis view: diastolic frame showing the aortic valve and the origin of the left main coronary artery
LMCA: left main coronary artery

C) *In M Mode*

The two aortic walls are visualised as two parallel echos defining the aortic lumen; they have an anterior motion in systole and a posterior motion in diastole (fig. 3-16)[131]. The internal diameter of the aorta ranges from 21 to 35 mm[239]. This measurement is taken at the onset of the QRS complex of the ECG,from the most anterior echo of the anterior wall to the most anterior echoe of the posterior wall of the aorta[174] (fig. 3-17). This diameter is slightly larger in systole than in diastole. The two parallel echos of the aortic wall define three separate cavities on the echocardiogram[239]; anteriorly, the outflow tract of the right ventricle, then the lumen of the aorta and posteriorly the left atrial cavity. As the aortic diameter varies with age and body surface area, it is convenient to use the ratio of left atrial diameter to aortic diameter which is normally just over 1 (LA/Ao $\simeq$ 1,1).[123] [171].

Fig. 3-16 Normal aortic
valve echogram
RCC: right coronary cusp
NCPC: non coronary
posterior cusp

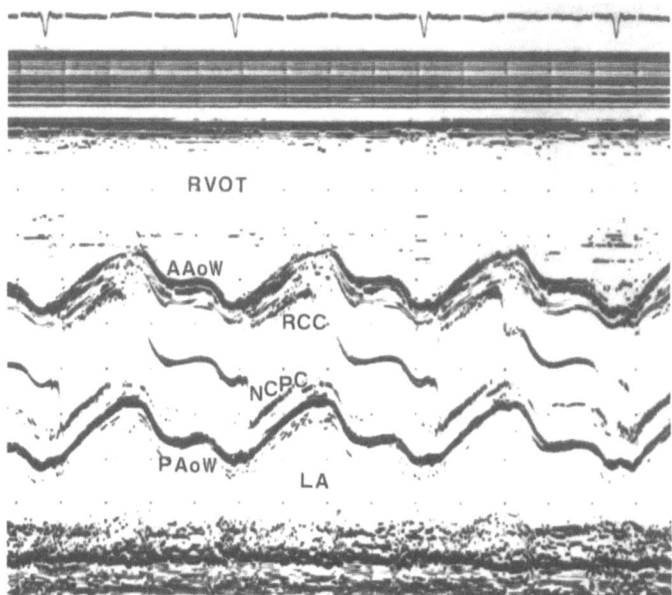

Fig. 3-17
The measurement of
systolic time intervals
from the aortic valve
echogram

PEP: preejection period
LVET: left ventricle
ejection time
ES: electromecanic time
⟷ separation of
the aortic leaflets
⟷ aortic root
diameter

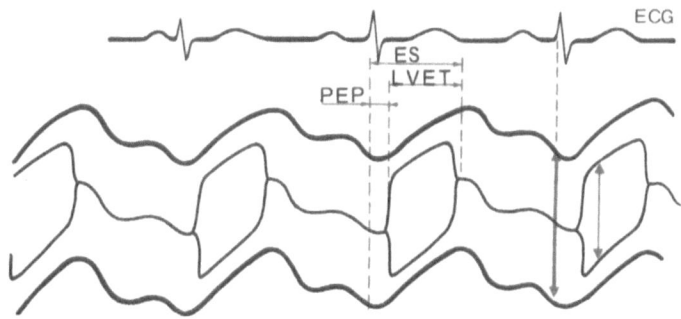

45

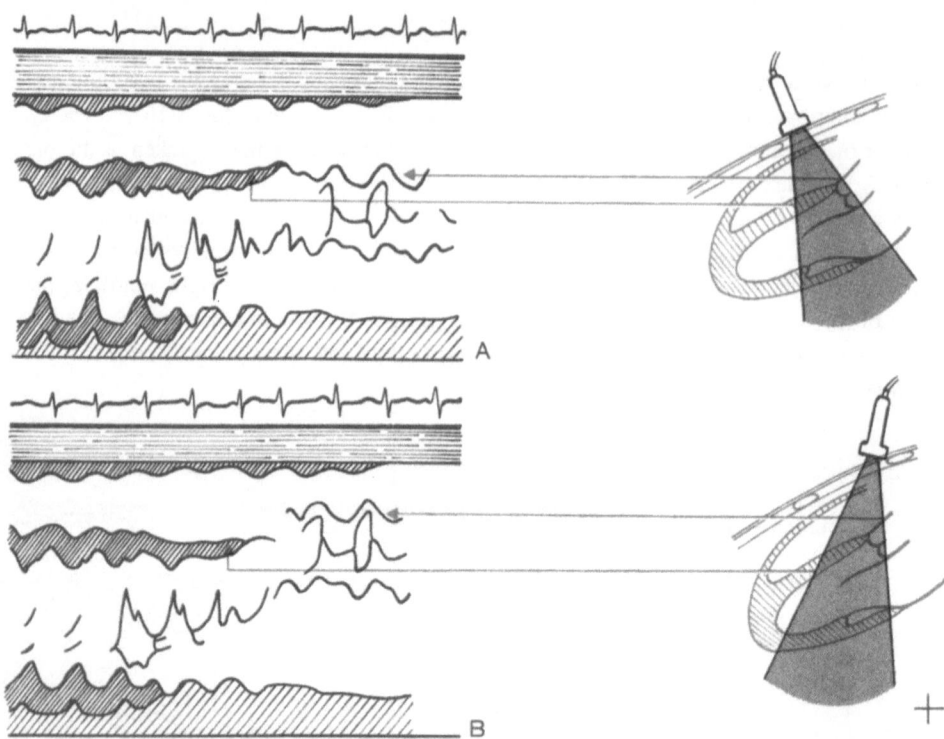

Fig.3-18 A- Normal continuity of the aortic and septal echos recorded with the transducer in the correct position

B- False overriding of the aorta produced by recording from a high intercostal space

By tilting the transducer caudally towards the mitral valve and left ventricle, the same aorto-septal and aorto-mitral continuity is observed[76]. Normally, the interventricular septum is located at the same level as the anterior aortic wall (fig.3-29), but if the position of the transducer on the chest wall is nearer the aorta than the septum, a false image of overriding aorta may be obtained (see Fallot's tetralogy).

In this case, the scan should be repeated with the transducer one, or even two, intercostal spaces lower (fig. 3-18).

· The echos of the aortic valve are recorded between the echos of the two aortic walls (fig. 3-17). They have a characteristic box-like appearance in systole, with a linear median echo in diastole[76]. The maximum separation of the anterior and posterior cusps is measured in early systole (normal = 16 to 25 mm)[239]. During systole, fine fluttering of the aortic cusps may be observed. The two cusps visualised, as in 2D, are the right coronary and the posterior non-coronary cusps (fig. 3-14)[131]. In recordings when the aortic valve echos are registred over several cardiac cycles, the systolic time intervals of the left ventricle may be measured. They correlate well with the values obtained by the traditional phonocardiographic methods with external pulse tracings[91].

The pre ejectional (PEP) and ejection (EP) periods and their ratio may therefore be measured (fig. 3-17).

46

3.1.3. Tricuspid Valve

The possibility of obtaining good views of the right heart chambers with 2D echocardiography allows detailed study of the tricuspid valve; only two of its leaflets are recorded at any one time.

A) 2D Long axis view

The tricuspid va've is usually recorded with the transducer in the left parasternal area tilted medially and saggitally (plate X)[200]. In practice, the apical and subcostal views give better images (fig. 3-19, plate VI, VIII).

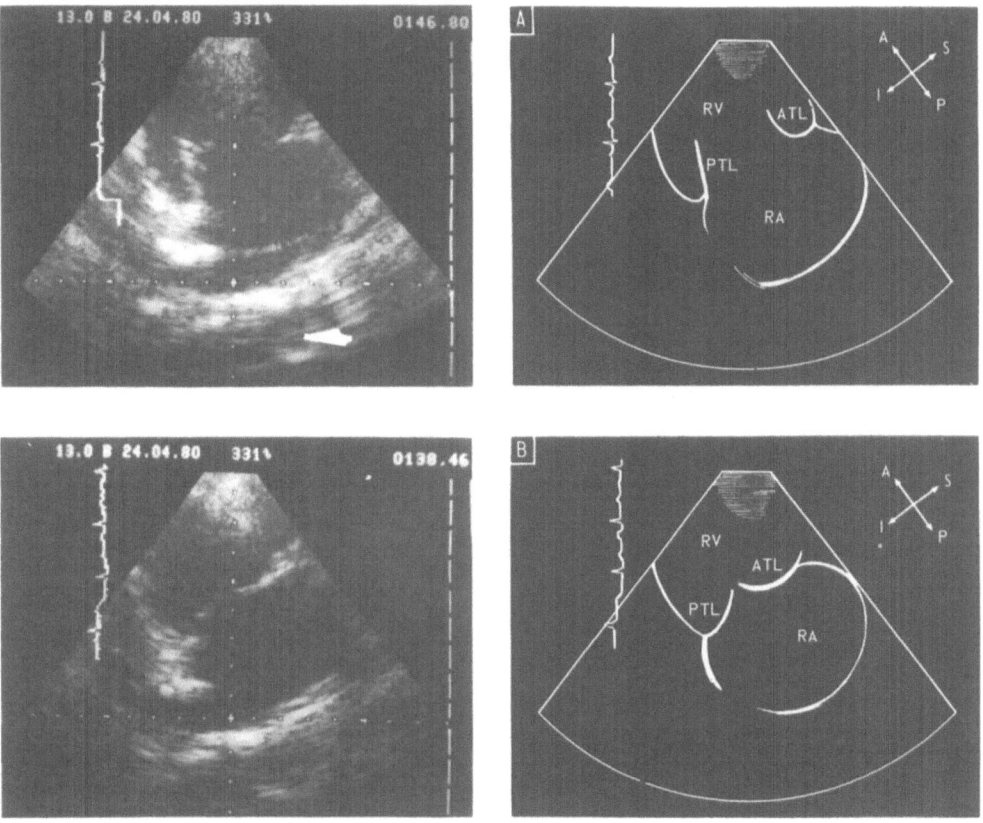

Fig. 3-19 2D parasternal long axis views of a normal tricuspid valve
A- Diastolic frame B- Systolic frame
PTL: posterior tricuspid leaflet
ATL: anterior tricuspid leaflet

The apical or four-chamber view visualises the anterior and septal leaflets and their insertion, located slightly closer to the apex than the mitral leaflets. The portion of the septum between the septal leaflets of the mitral and tricuspid valves defines the anatomical relationship of the left ventricle and the right atrium (membranous septum)[54] [200] (fig 3-38, plate VI).

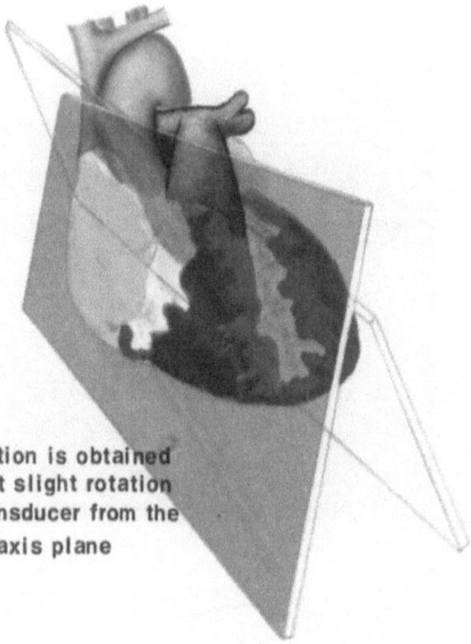

This section is obtained by a right slight rotation of the transducer from the long axis plane

Anatomic drawing

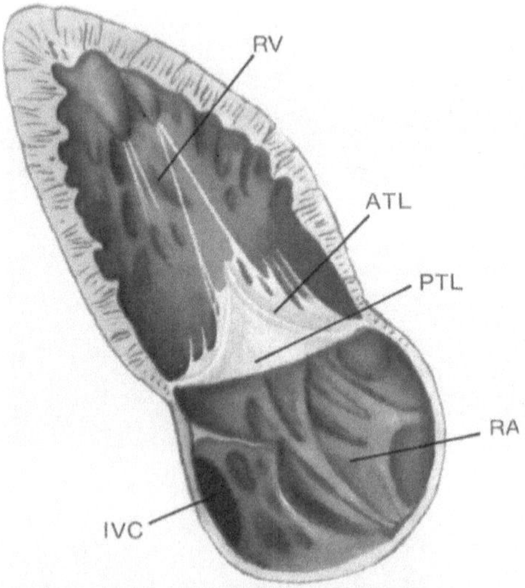
RV
ATL
PTL
RA
IVC

2D ECHO

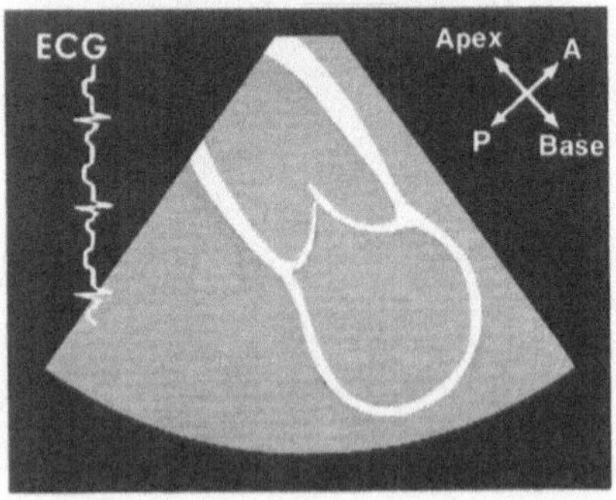
ECG
Apex
A
P
Base

Tardieu

The subcostal view gives a good appreciation of the tricuspid ring and its chordae tendinae.

B) *Short axis view*

This is usually recorded near the base of the heart, where the septal and anterior tricuspid leaflets are visualised to the left of the aorta[200]. They have an anterior diastolic motion (fig. 3-20).

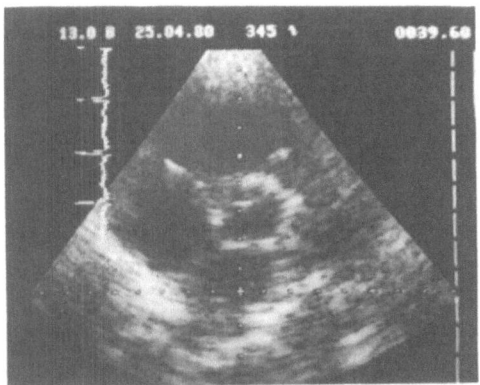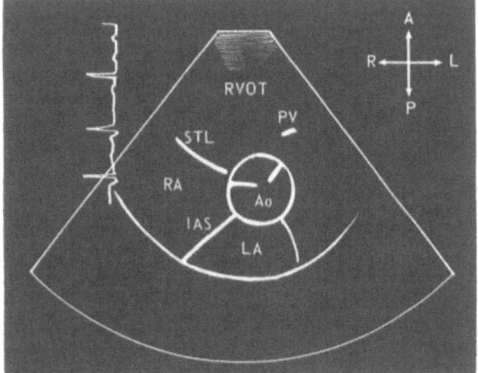

Fig. 3-20 2D parasternal short axis view. Diastolic frame showing a normal tricuspid valve.
STL: septal tricuspid leaflet

C) *M Mode*

The M mode appearances are usually limited to the recording of the early diastolic opening of the anterior or septal leaflets (fig. 3-21)[54] [130]. When it is possible to record them throughout the whole of diastole, their motion resembles that of the mitral valve but they remain anterior to the ventricular septum (fig. 3-29)[178].

The leaflet has an anterior motion in early diastole, tends to close in mid diastole and then reopens with atrial contraction. The same phases than for the mitral valve with D, E, F, A; B, C, points may be defined (fig. 3-22) The tricuspid EF slope has a normal value of between 60 and 125 mm/sec. Occasionally, the posterior tricuspid leaflet may be identified and, as with the posterior mitral leaflet, it appears as a mirror image of smaller amplitude of the anterior leaflet[178]. It must be emphasised that the tricuspid valve is easier to record when the right ventricle is dilated. Scanning shows the continuity of the septal tricuspid leaflet and the anterior wall of the aorta (fig. 3-23).

3.1.4. Pulmonary Valve

This is one of the most difficult structures to record in M mode. However, it is easier to locate in 2D and its motion may be analysed by simultaneous M mode recording. It is only visualised in the transverse view. (plate V, fig 3-20)

Usually, only the posterior cusp is recorded. It is a fine, mobile echoe situated anteriorly and to the right of the aorta. It may also be recorded from the subcostal area (plate IX).

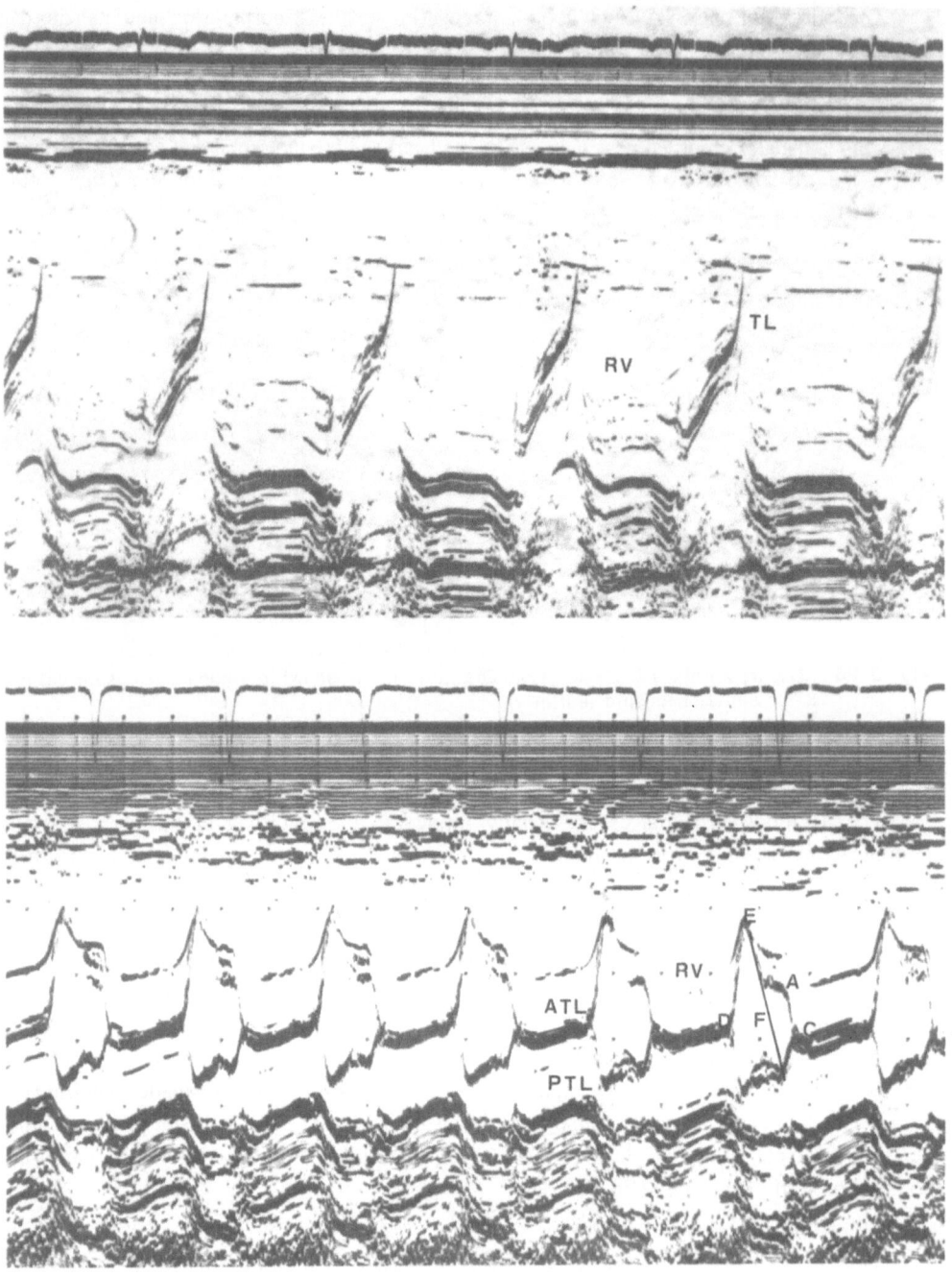

Fig. 3-21 **Fig. 3-22**   Normal tricuspid valve echogram
TL: tricuspid leaflet
ATL: anterior tricuspid leaflet
PTL: posterior tricuspid leaflet

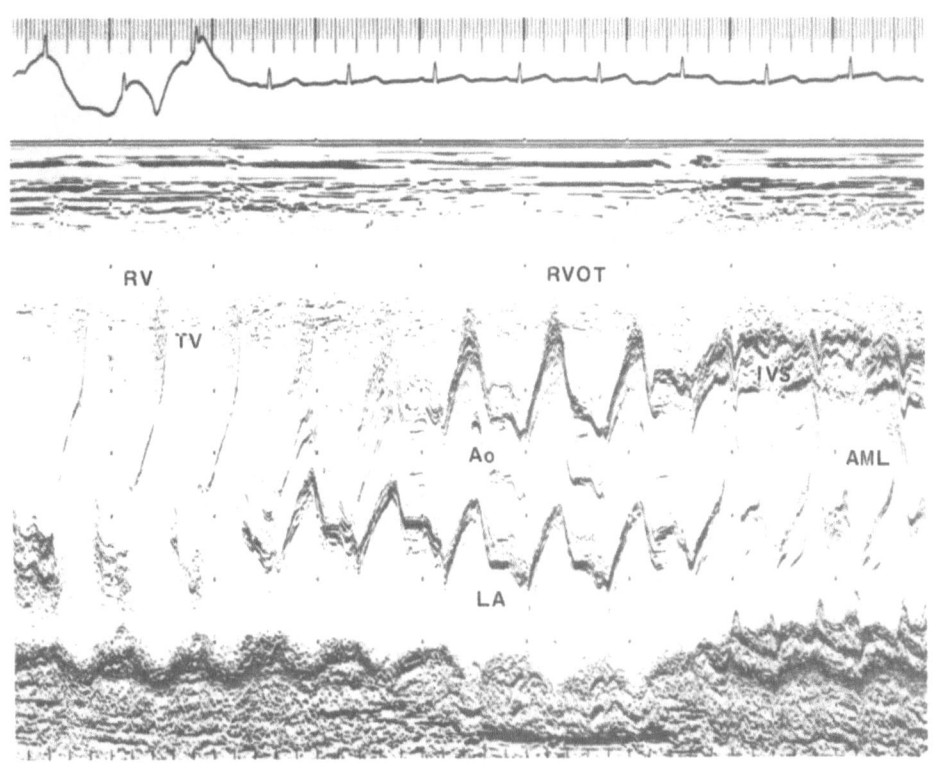

Fig. 3-23 Normal tricuspid valve M mode scan showing the relative positions of the tricuspid, aortic and mitral valves

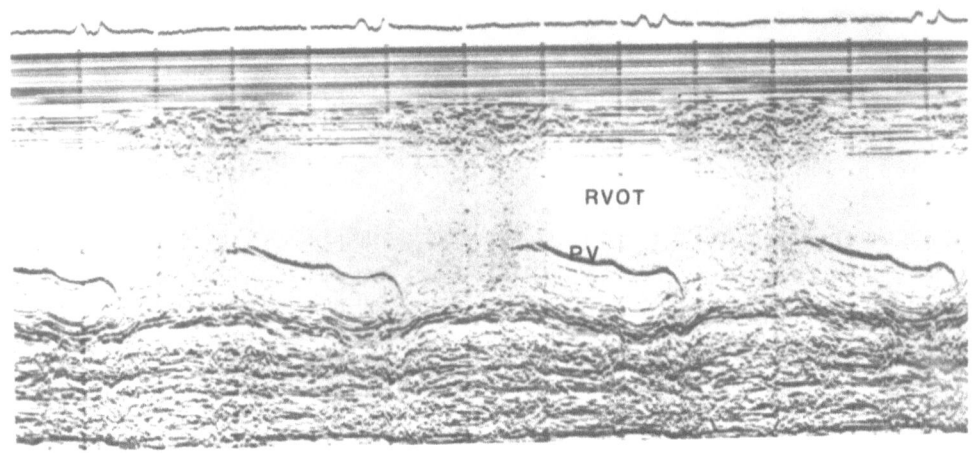

Fig. 3-24 Normal pulmonary valve echogram

In M mode (fig. 3-24), the pulmonary valve is located at the junction of the right ventricular outflow tract and the pulmonary artery (fig. 3-28, 3-29). Usually, only the

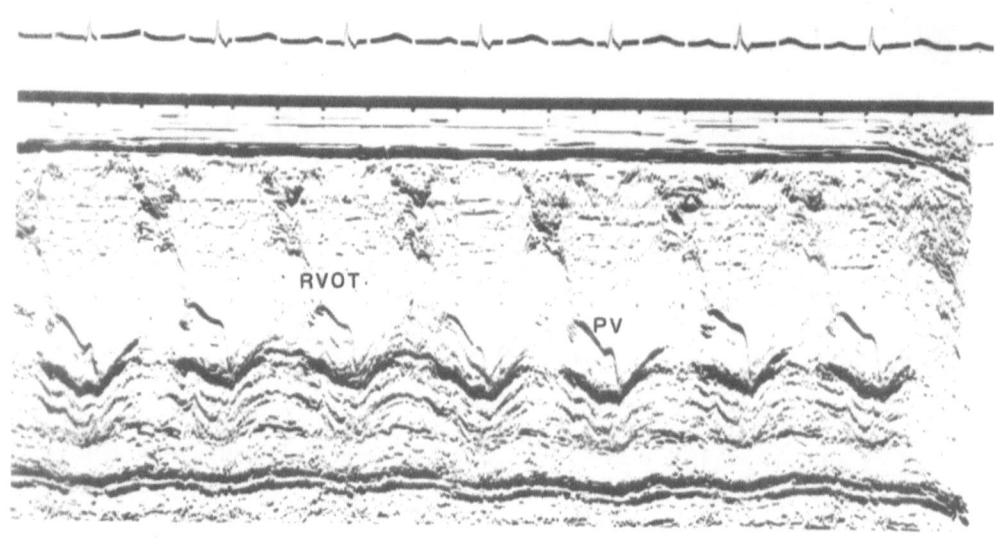

Fig. 3-25 Pulmonary valve echogram showing variation in the depth of the "A" wave with respiration

Fig.3-26
Pulmonary valve echogram
showing the anterior and
posterior pulmonary
leaflets with their
"box-like" appearance
in systole.

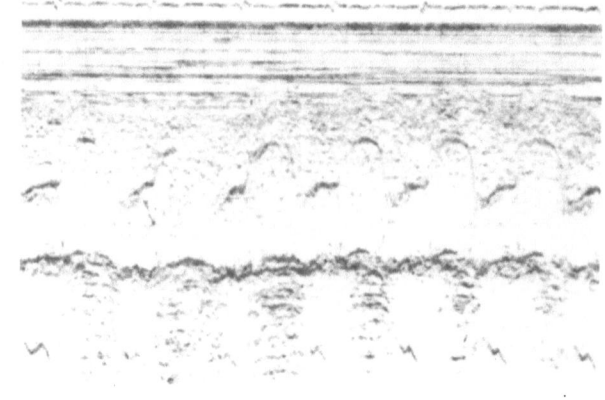

posterior cusp is recorded[131]. It has a sloping, linear diastolic echoe, located in the middle of the pulmonary infundibulum. Atrial systole causes a small posterior motion just before systolic opening. The amplitude of this A wave is about 3 mm but there is some respiratory variation (fig. 3-25)[223]. At the onset of right ventricular systole the valve opens with a rapid posterior motion of about 300 mm/sec[145]. The echoe is seldom recorded throughout systole[54]. Rarely, the anterior pulmonary leaflet is recorded simultaneously, giving the same "box-like" appearance as the systolic phase of the aortic valve (fig. 3-26).

The right ventricular systolic time intervals may be measured[91]. The ratio of the pre-ejection period (PEP) to the right ventricular ejection time (RVET) is a good index of right ventricular function (fig. 3-27).

The echocardiographic assessment of these indices gives useful information, which can otherwise only be obtained by invasive haemodynamic investigations.

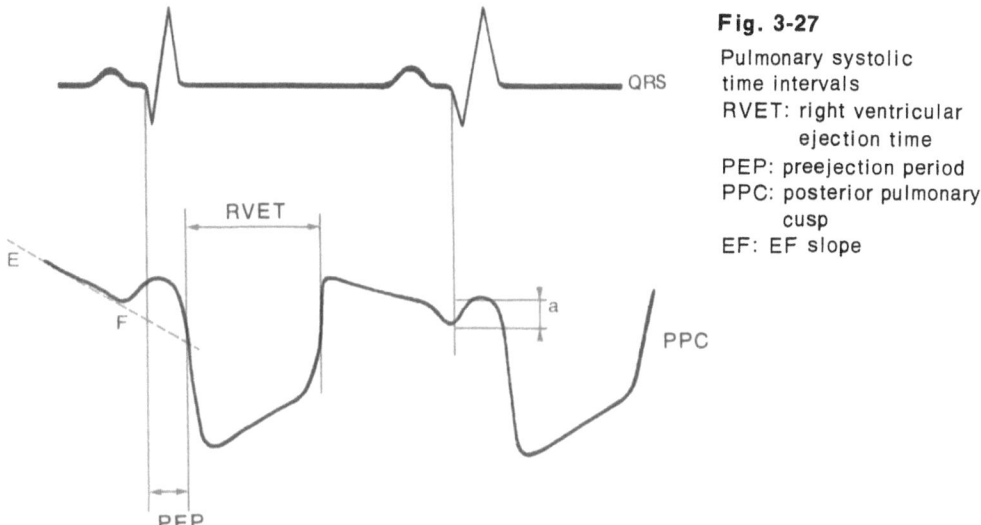

Fig. 3-27

Pulmonary systolic
time intervals
RVET: right ventricular
ejection time
PEP: preejection period
PPC: posterior pulmonary
cusp
EF: EF slope

Fig. 3-28

M mode scan from the pulmonary
valve to the aorta

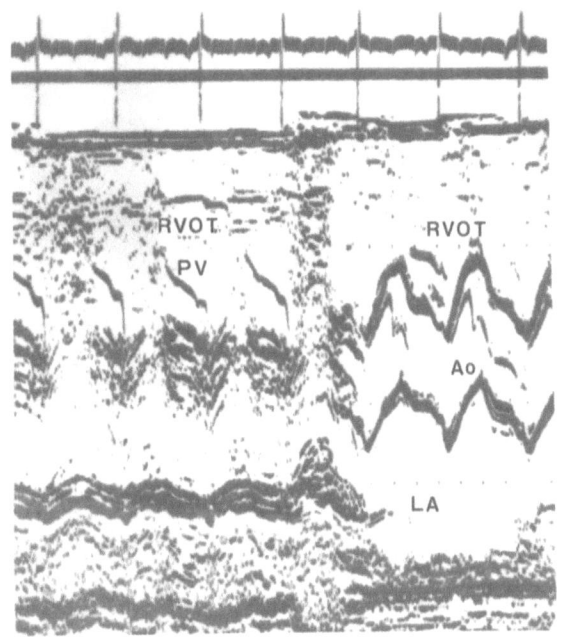

3.2 CARDIAC CAVITIES

A series of dense linear echos 2-4 cm wide, anteriór to the heart are recorded with the transducer in the left parasternal region. They correspond to the chest wall, a structure which is in direct contact with the anterior wall of the right ventricle.

3.2.1. Right Heart

The form of the right ventricle (RV) is complex. It partially surrounds the left ventricle

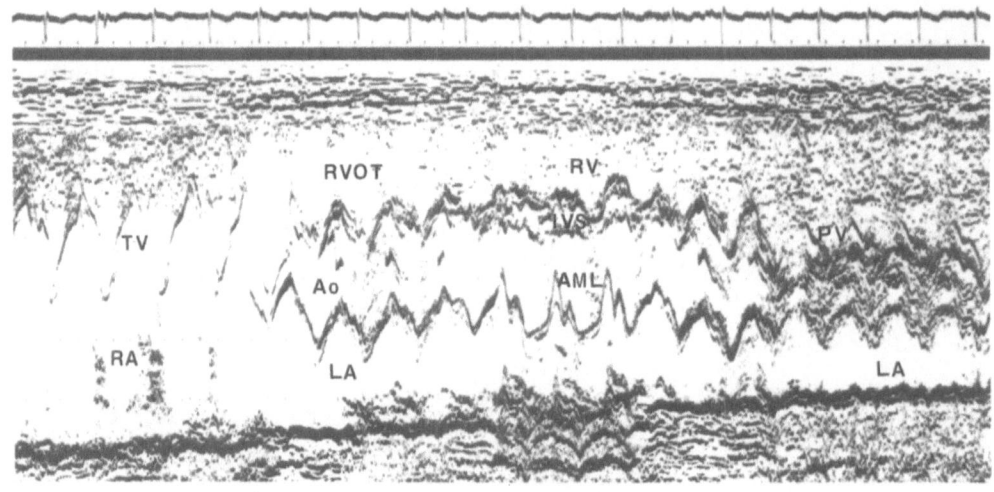

Fig. 3-29 M mode scan showing the relative positions of the four cardiac valves
TV: tricuspid valve   Ao: aortic valve
AML: anterior mitral leaflet   PV: pulmonary valve

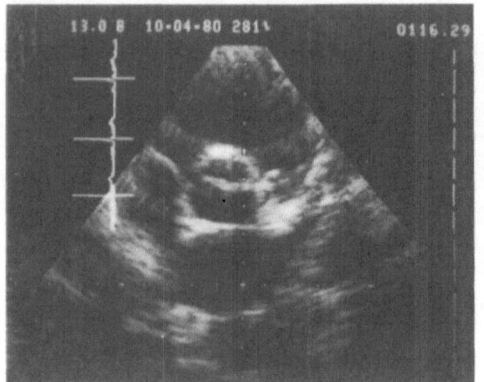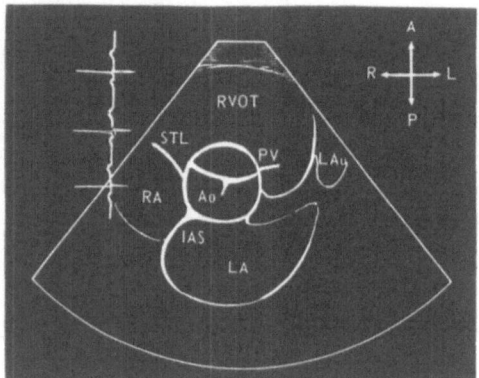

Fig. 3-30 2D short axis view through the right atrium (RA), the septal tricuspid leaflet (STL), the right ventricular outflow tract (RVOT) and pulmonary valve (PV). LAu: left auricle

and, only by examination in a number of planes, can its geometry be studied. This is the great advantage of 2D over M mode echo. The right heart is more completely visualised, especially the right atrium (RA) which can only be definitely identified by this technique[177] [200].

A) *Long axis*

In the usual parasternal position (plate II), only the anterior portion of the RV and the pulmonary infundibulum are visible. Angling the transducer medially in the true sagittal plane (plate X) a view of the RV, tricuspid valve and RA may be obtained together with the anterior wall of the RV[200] (fig. 3-19).

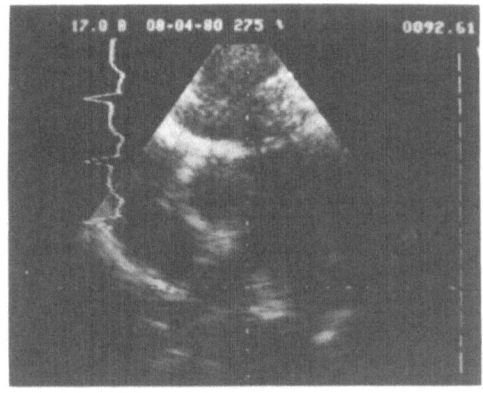
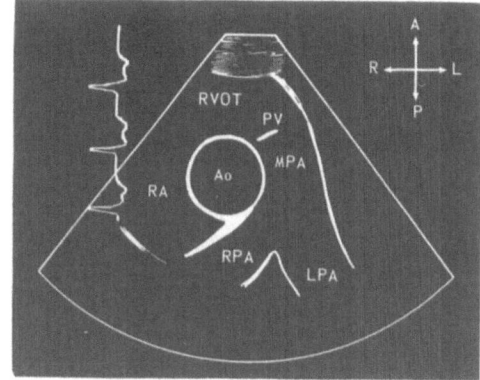

Fig. 3-31   2D short axis parasternal view showing the bifurcation of the main
pulmonary artery (MPA)
RPA: right pulmonary artery
LPA: left pulmonary artery

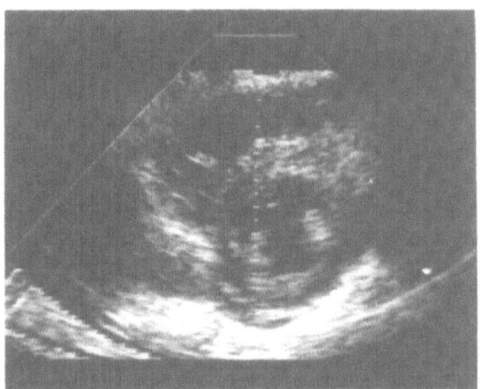
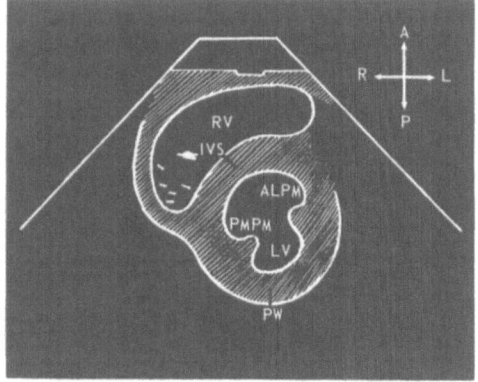

*****Fig. 3-32** 2D short axis view through the mitral papillary muscles. Note the crescent shape
of the right ventricle around the left ventricular chamber
PMPM: postero-medial papillary muscle
ALPM: antero-lateral papillary muscle

In the apical 4-chamber view the two ventricles are recorded simultaneously along their
long axes, separated by the interventricular septum. The two atria and the interatrial septum
are visualised posteriorly[13] [177] [200].

In this incidence, the apical and lateral walls of the RV may be studied.

The 4-chamber view may also be obtained from the subcostal area (plate VIII) but in this
case the infero-diaphragmatic wall of the RV is visualised[200] (fig. 3-40).

B) *Short axis view*

In the parasternal area, the short axis view at aortic level shows the pulmonary
infundibulum circling around the aorta and continuing as the main pulmonary artery (plate V,
fig. 3-30); by angling the transducer, the pulmonary artery may be followed to its

bifurcation[173] [200] (fig. 3-31). The RA is situated behind the tricuspid valve. Apical scanning gives a series of sections through the RV and shows its "crescent-like" shape around the

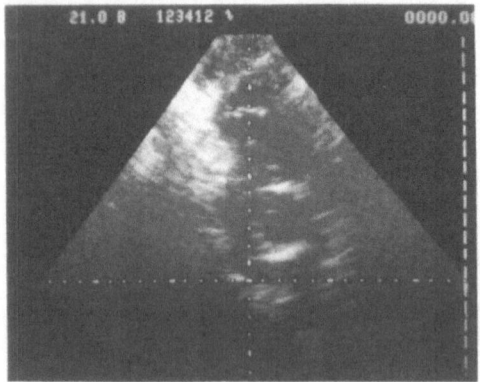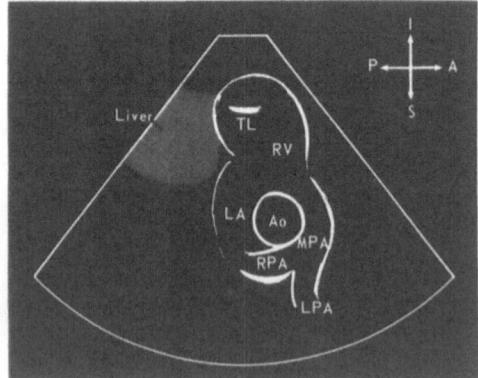

Fig. 3-33 2D subcostal view showing the bifurcation of the main pulmonary artery (MPA)
RPA: right pulmonary artery
LPA: left pulmonary artery

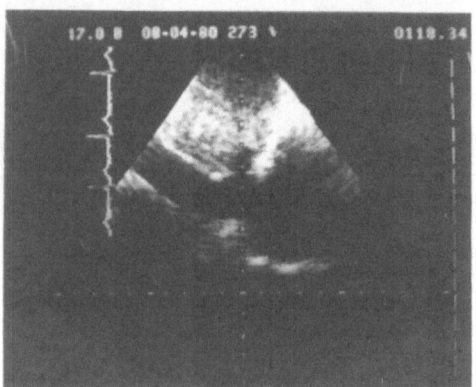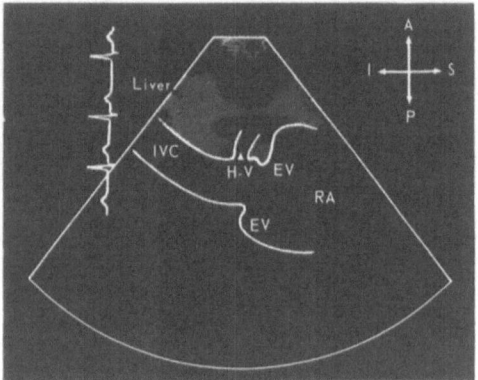

Fig. 3-34 2D subcostal view of a dilated inferior vena cava
IVC: inferior vena cava
EV: Eustachi's valve
HV: hepatic vein

LV[104] (fig. 3-32, plate III). The same appearances may be recorded from the subcostal position by rotating the transducer 90° with respect to the 4-chamber-view[200]. Scanning towards the base of the heart shows the pulmonary infundibulum encircling the aorta and the RA (fig. 3-33). By orientating the beam towards the abdomen, the inferior vena cava (IVC) (fig. 3-34) and its arrival in the RA with the Eustachian valve and the hepatic veins may be recorded[124]. The internal dimension of the IVC varies with the respiratory cycle, decreasing during inspiration. This distinguishes it from the abdominal aorta.

The anterior chamber in the left parasternal area corresponds to the RV. This chamber is studied in the so called routine ventricular incidence. The anterior wall echos lie under the chest wall. It is about 4 mm thick in adults, and it presents a posterior motion during systolic contraction. The right ventricular internal dimension is measured from the internal edge of the anterior wall to the right border of the interventricular septum[54] [174]. This dimension is taken in the supine position (it being increased to a variable degree in the left lateral position) at the onset of QRS. The normal range lies between 8 and 17 mm[160], depending on the body surface area (see Appendix). The right ventricle may vary physiologically with respiration (increase of 2-3 mm during inspiration), and there is a great deal of individual variation. Therefore, it is better to use the ratio of the right to left ventricular end diastolic internal dimension (RV/LV)[118], which is normally 0,33 for all ages, rather than make an exact measurement (except for newborn). In all cases, the definition of the anterior wall and septal echos requires careful adjustment of the near gain and time gain compensation[54]. The pulmonary infundibulum, visualised by scanning in the aortic incidence, has the same dimension as that of the aorta (fig. 3-29).

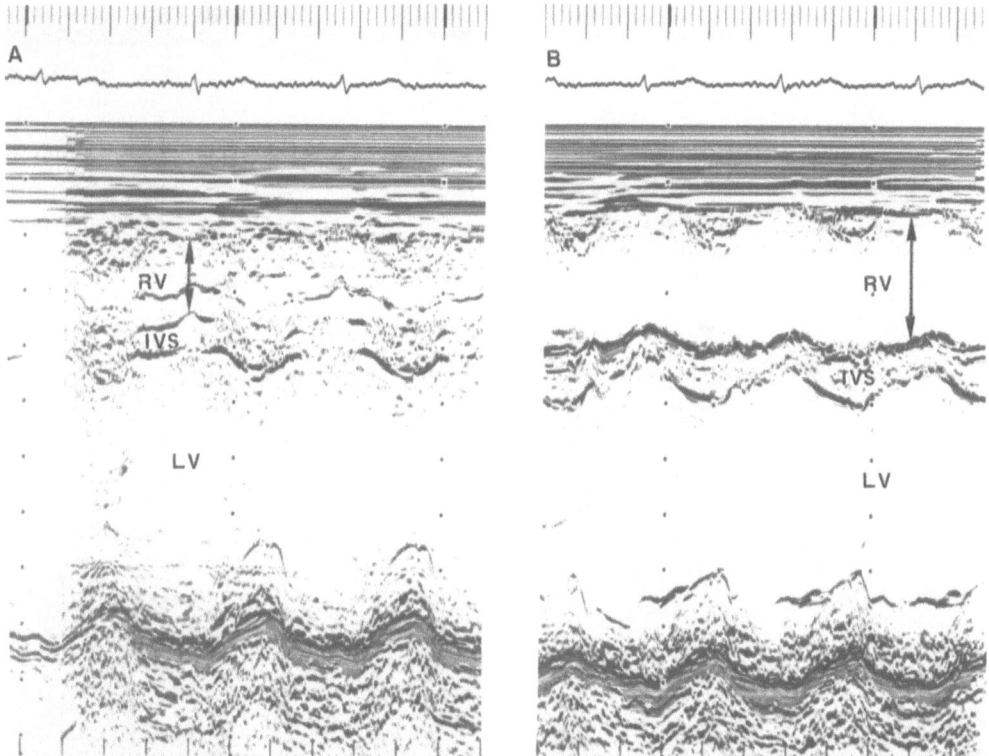

Fig. 3-35 Right ventricular internal diameter in the same patient
A- Supine: 12 mm; the definition of the interventricular septum is poor
B- Left lateral: the quality of the second has improved but the RV internal diameter has increased significantly (22 mm)

3.2.2. Left heart

The interventricular septum will be treated with the left ventricle (LV) as, normally, it participates in left ventricular ejection and the interatrial septum with the left atrium (LA).

A) *Long axis* (plate II, fig. 3-36)

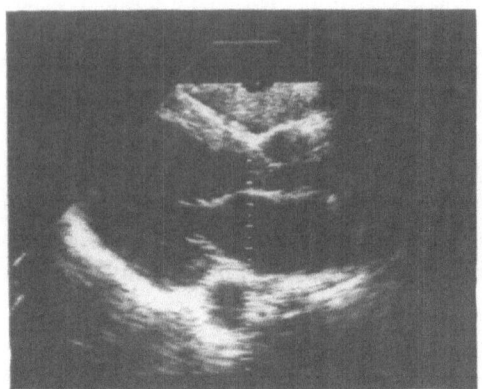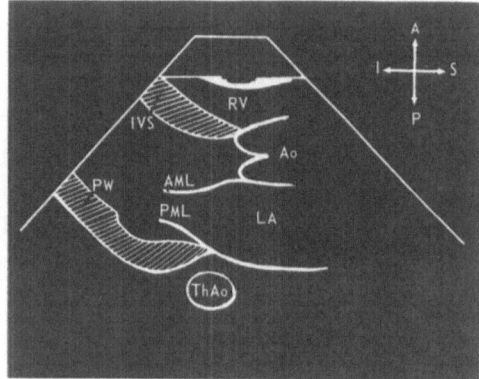

* **Fig. 3-36** 2D parasternal long axis diastolic frame

In the parasternal position, the anterior portion of the interventricular septum is visualised all along its length from this origin at the anterior wall of the aorta. These two structures are usually in the same plane, but when the heart lies horizontally the septum bulges anteriorly and forms and obtuse angle with the aorta (fig. 3-37).

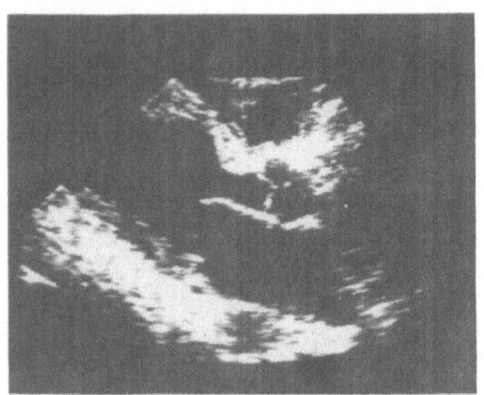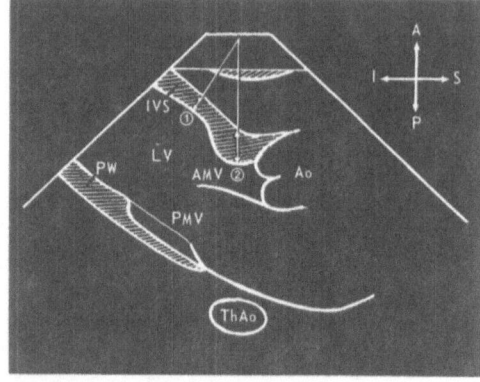

* **Fig. 3-37** 2D parasternal long axis view. M mode recording in position (1) would record the true thickness of the interventricular septum.
In position (2) the septal thickness would be exaggerated giving a false impression of subaortic septal hypertrophy

The left ventricle is recorded in its long axis, at least as far as the insertion of the posteromedial papillary muscles, the apex being poorly defined[54] [177] [200]. The LA is situated behind the aorta; its anteroposterior dimension may be measured.

The apical position gives priviledged views of the LV, as much of the chamber may be visualised by rotating the transducer around the long axis[177] [200].

In the so-called 4-chamber view, the mid-part of the septum (junction of the anterior and posterior or inferior portions), the apex and lateral walls may be examined. The LA lies behind the mitral valve taken in an infero-superior axis. The pulmonary veins may generally be identified[175]. The interatrial septum follows on from the membranous part of the interventricular septum. Occasionally, a break in continuity at the level of the fossa ovale is observed but this does not imply the presence of an atrial septal defect[177] (plate VI, fig. 3-38).

By rotating the transducer 90°, an image equivalent of the right anterior oblique view on angiography is obtained. The anterior, apical and inferior walls can then be studied[177] (plate VII, fig. 3-39).

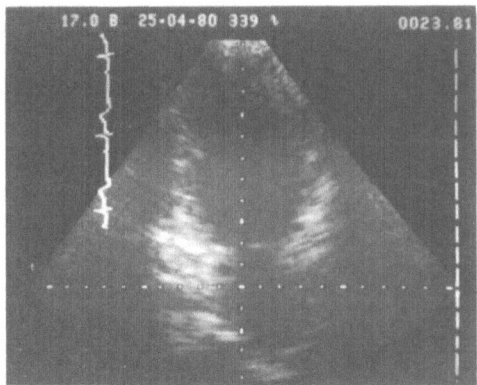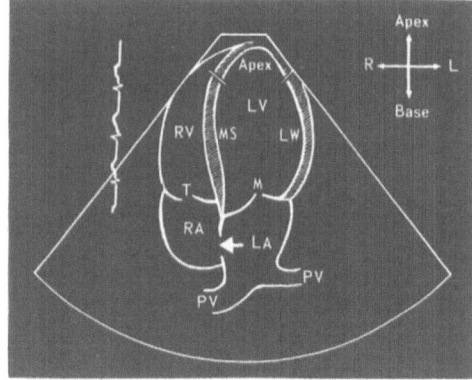

Fig. 3-38 2D apical 4 chamber view. The pulmonary veins are recorded draining into the left atrium. The foramen ovale is shown (arrow).
MS: middle septum   LW: lateral wall
PV : pulmonary vein

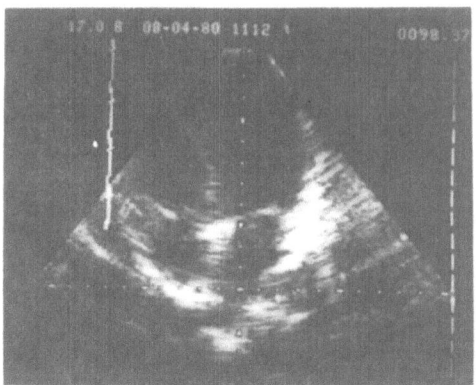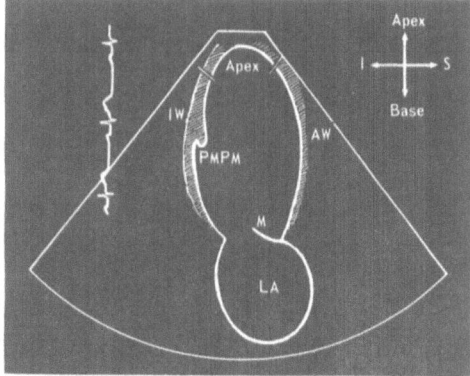

Fig. 3-39 2D apical "pseudo-RAO" view at 90° to the normal 4 chamber view
AW: anterior wall   PMPM: postero-medial papillary muscle
IW: inferior wall

In the subcostal 4-chamber view (plate VIII, fig. 3-40), the inferior portion of the interventricular septum and the anterolateral wall are viewed[200]. This is the best incidence for studying the interatrial septum which normally bulges into the RA in systole[10]. Simultaneous M mode recording allows detailed analysis of its motion throughout the cardiac cycle (fig. 3-41).

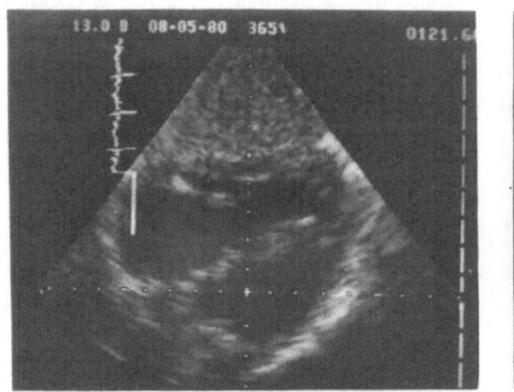 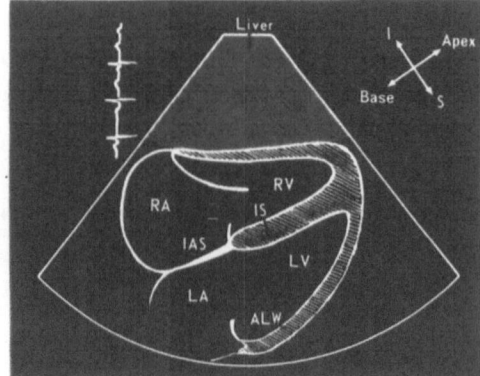

Fig: 3-40 2D subcostal 4 chamber view
ALW: antero-lateral wall
IAS: interatrial septum

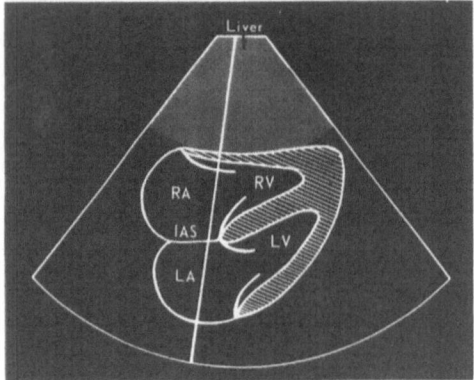

TM line on the IAS

Fig. 3-41
Diagram showing the method for M mode recording of the interatrial septum

Normal M mode appearance
of the interatrial septum ▶

B) Short axis views

In the left parasternal position, the transverse view through the base of the heart (plate V) sections the LA through its short axis posterior to the aorta[41] [54] (fig. 3-30).

60

The left ventricle may be studied in detail by scanning down towards the apex; the left ventricular outflow tract (plate IV, fig. 3-42), the short axis (plate III, fig. 3-43) and the papillary muscles (fig. 3-44). The short axis may be considered the equivalent of the left anterior oblique angiographic view of the left ventricle[177] [179].

The following walls are visualised, the length of the interventricular septum, concave towards the left ventricle and the inferior, anterior and lateral walls. To the apex, two muscular projections corresponding to the postero-medial and antero-lateral papillary muscles of the mitral valve are observed[140]. The same short axis views of the LV may sometimes be recorded from the subcostal position (fig. 3-45).

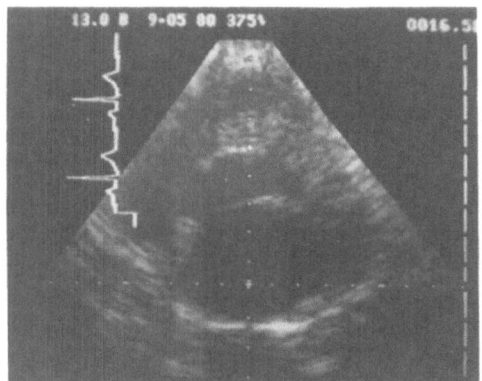 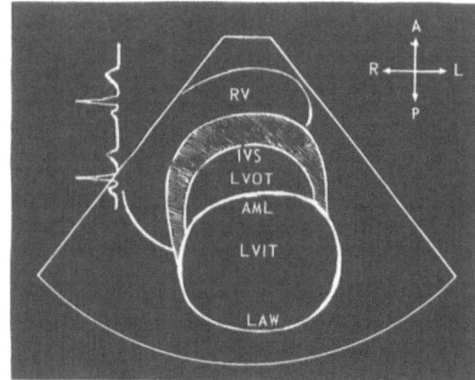

Fig. 3-42 2D parasternal short axis (n° 3) view
LVOT: LV outflow tract
LVIT: LV inflow tract

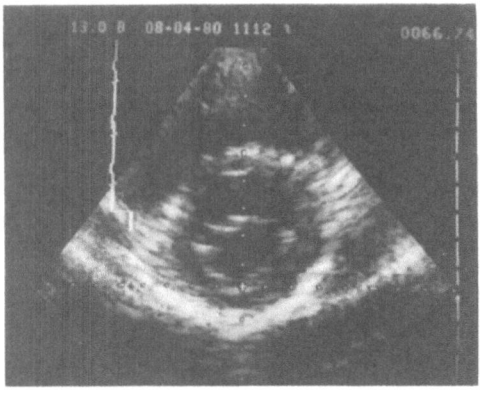 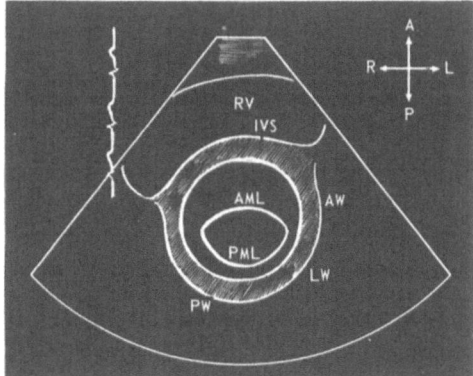

Fig. 3-43 2D parasternal short axis view corresponding to the LAO projection

61

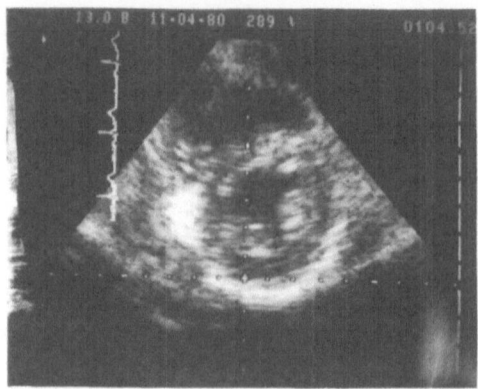
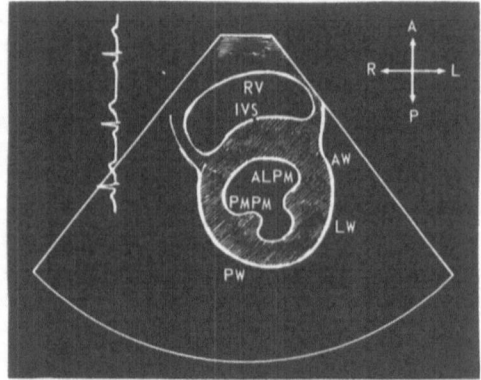

Fig. 3-44 2D parasternal short axis (n° 1) view
AW: anterior wall   ALPM: antero-lateral papillary muscle
PMPM: postero-medial papillary muscle

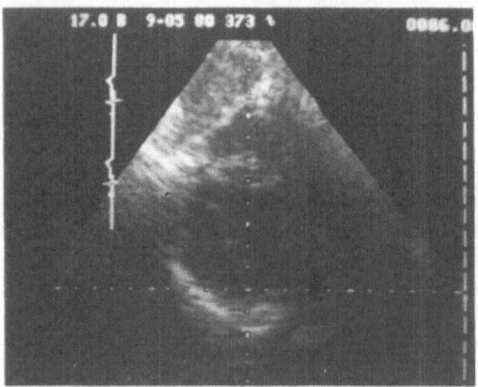
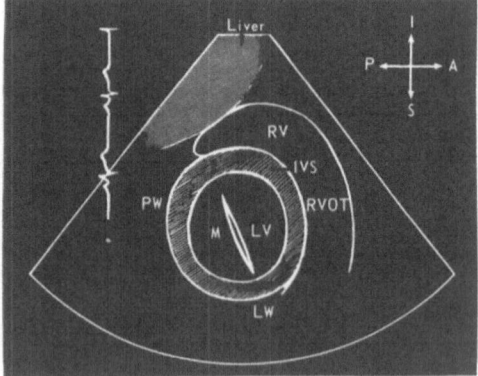

Fig. 3-45 2D subcostal short axis (n° 2) view

C) *M mode study of the left heart*

This analysis is performed from the left parasternal position by scanning from the base towards the apex (plate II, fig. 3-46).

— *LA*

The LA is located posterior to the aorta at the base of the heart. The M mode recording may be divided into three separate regions of about the same size (fig. 3-16).

By convention, the internal dimension is measured in early diastole when its diameter is maximal: this is the antero-postero dimension from the posterior wall of the aorta to the left atrial posterior wall[90]. In adults, this is usually about 30 mm but often the LA/AO ratio is used which is normally about 1,1[166]. The internal dimension varies during the cardiac cycle and some workers[196] have suggested an index of left ventricular filling based on the motion of the posterior aortic wall (fig. 3-47).

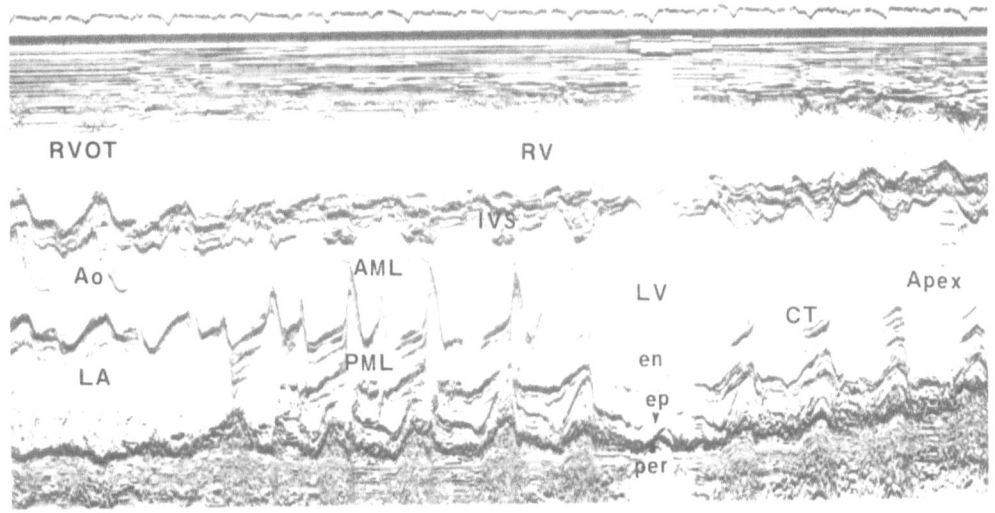

Fig. 3-46 M mode scan showing the ideal incidence ⇕ for measurement of the left
ventricular internal dimensions
en: endocardium
ep: epicardium
per: pericardium

Scanning down towards the apex brings the LA posterior wall into view behind the anterior mitral leaflet. It shows an anterior diastolic motion starting with the onset of the P wave on the ECG (fig. 3-48). Its echo is in continuity with that of the posterior mitral leaflet and the left ventricular posterior wall (fig. 3-46).

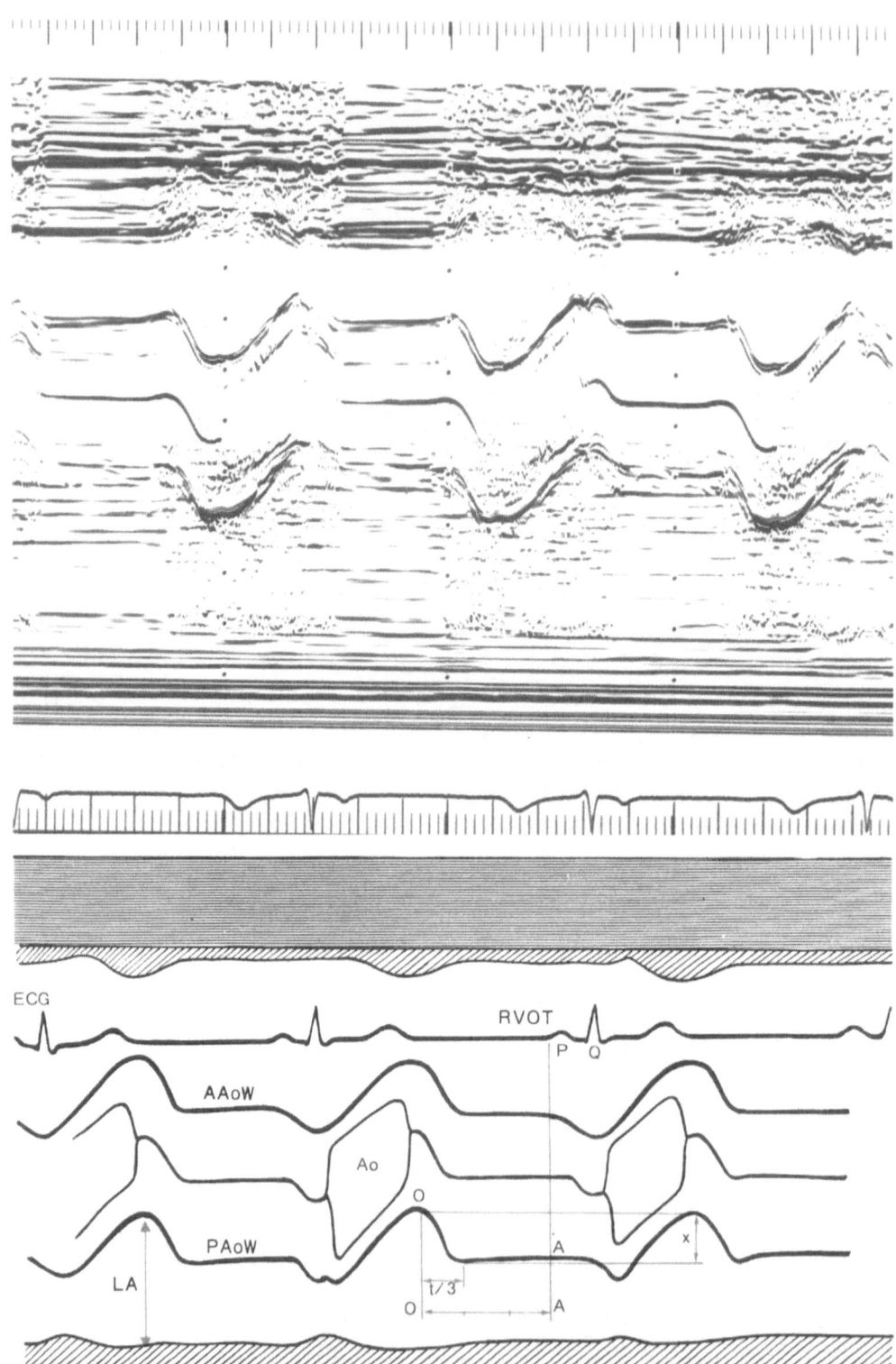

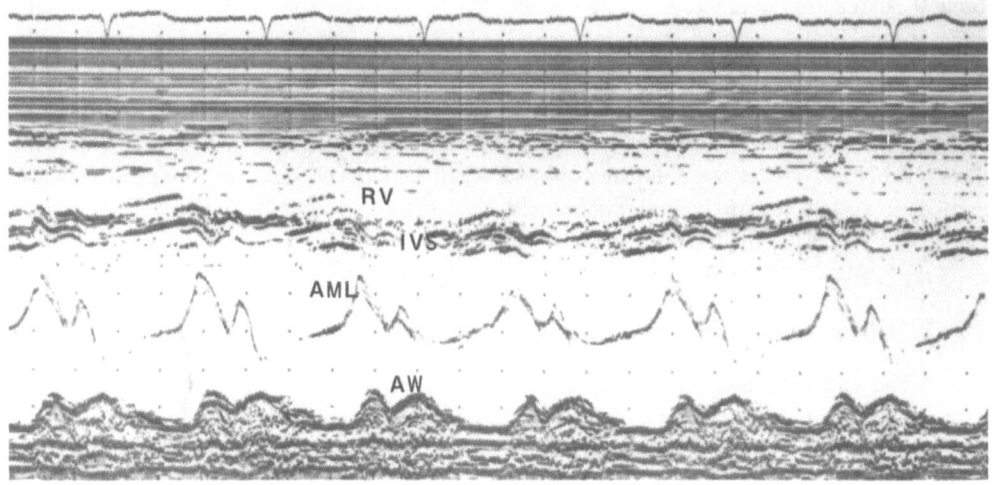

Fig. 3-48 M mode recording showing the posterior left atrial wall (AW) behind the anterior mitral leaflet (AML)   AW: atrial wall

— LV

M mode study of the LV implies good quality recordings in order to obtain reliable repetitive measurements; these measurements are always taken in the so-called routine position (Feigenbaum's position 2) which visualises the free edges of the mitral valves and the chordae[54]. This is the antero-posterior short axis of the LV[68] [81] [166] (fig. 3-49).

Recording with the patient slightly turned on his left side often gives a better definition of the parietal echos without changing the values of the left ventricular dimensions significantly[7].

The septum and posterior wall move towards the left ventricular cavity during systole and both participate in its systolic shortening.

The diastolic dimension is measured at the onset of QRS from the left edge of the septum to the endocardial echo of the left ventricular posterior wall. The normal adult value averages 46 ± 4 mm[7]. The systolic internal dimension is measured at the end of systole and is defined as the shortest distance between the left edge of the septum and the endocardium of the posterior wall. The motion and the thickness of each of these walls are analysed.

— Septum [1] (fig. 3-49, 3-50)

The proximal subaortic 1/3 of the septum has a motion which is related to that of the aorta and therefore it should not be studied in this region[86]. In the routine LV position the mid third of the anterior septum is viewed. It has a posterior systolic motion of 4-5 mm which lasts

Fig. 3-47   Index of left atrial emptying $\dfrac{x}{1/3\,OA}$ $0,9 < n < 1$

This index is obtained by dividing the excursion x of the aorta dwing the first 1/3 of atrial emptying by the period OA corresponding to the duration of passive left ventricular filling about 0,30 sec. Its contraction finishes before that of the posterior wall. An early diastolic notch is commonly recorded at the left septal border, contemporary to aortic valve closure[54]; this is followed by anterior diastolic motion during the rapid left ventricular filling phase. In late diastole a small anterior displacement is observed due to atrial contraction. Its diastolic thickness is measured from the most anterior echo of its right border to the most anterior echo of its left border. The average thickness in adults is 8-9 mm. The same measurement may also be made in systole at its maximum thickness[42].

— *Posterior wall* (fig. 3-49).

Definition of the limits of the left ventricular posterior wall is often difficult.

• The endocardium which is a fine structure must not be confused with echos arising from chordae which are situated more anteriorly. They may be distinguished by their continuity with the echos of the mitral leaflets and by the absence of a posterior end-diastolic motion.

• The epicardium is recognised by the use of damping or switch gain controls. It may be distinguished from the pericardium, a denser echo, from which it may be separated by a small echo free space in systole[54] (fig. 3-46). The posterior wall moves anteriorly in systole with an

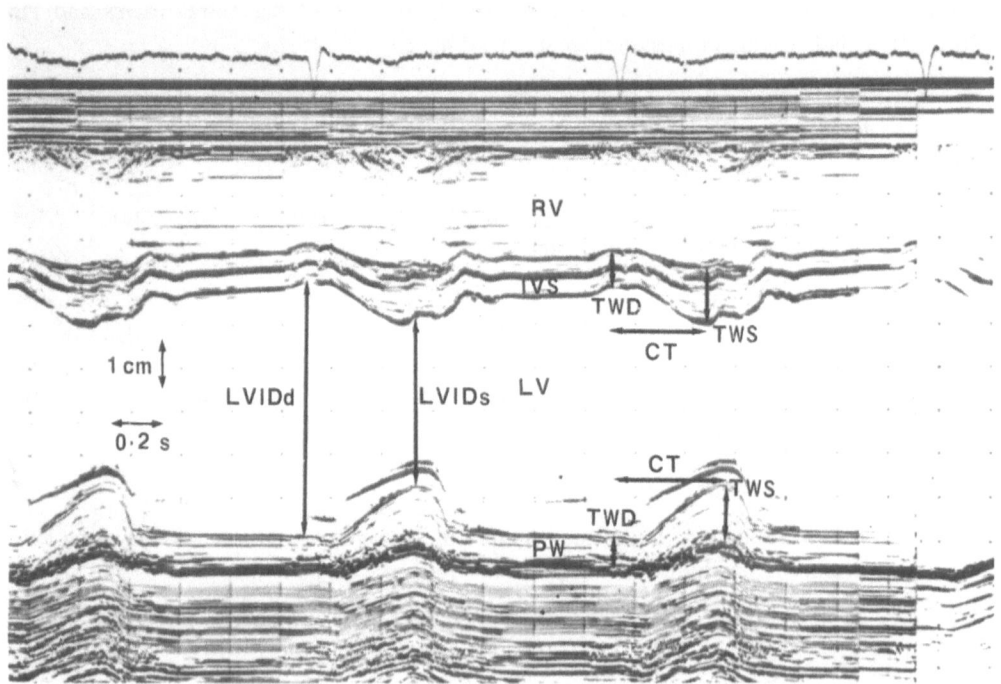

Fig. 3-49 Measurement of left ventricular internal dimensions and wall thickness
LVID : left ventricle internal diameter d: diastolic s: systolic
TW: thickness wall
CT: contraction time

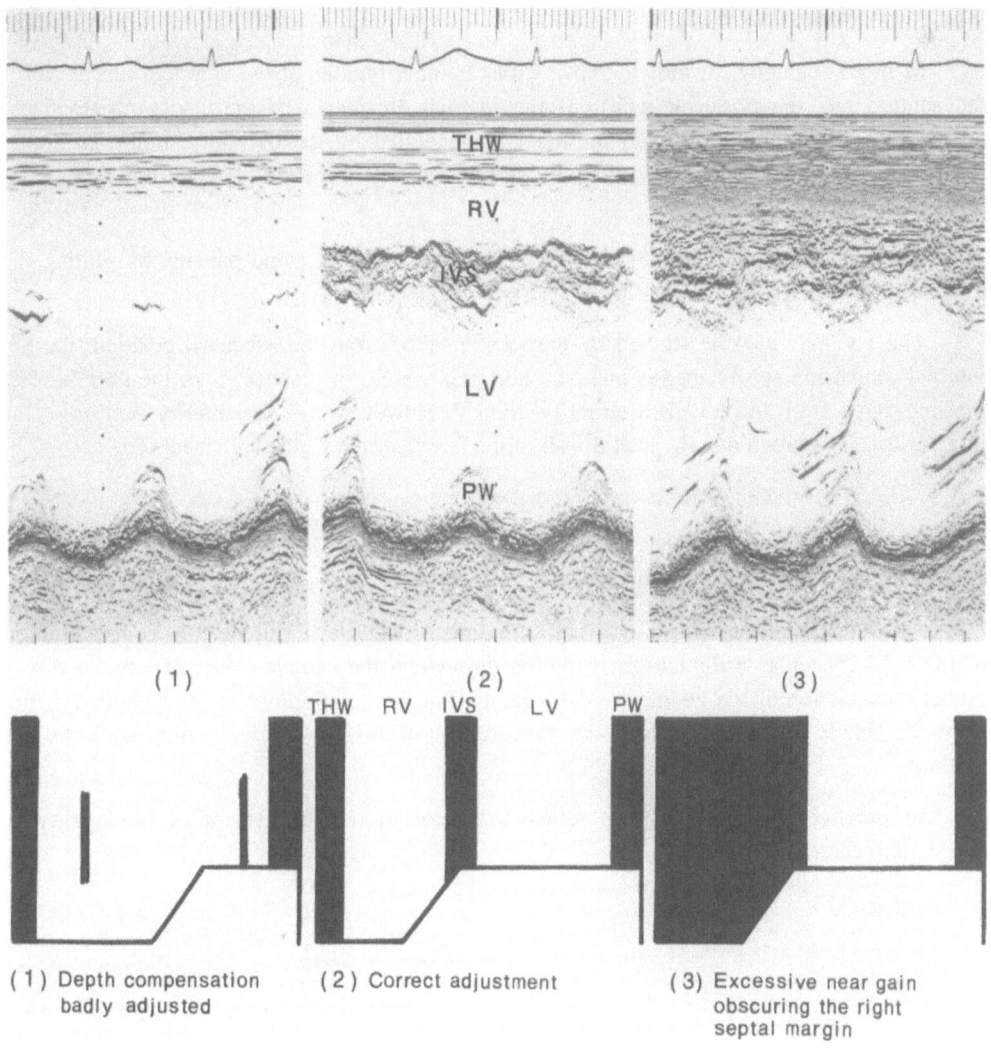

(1) Depth compensation badly adjusted

(2) Correct adjustment

(3) Excessive near gain obscuring the right septal margin

Fig. 3-50 Adjustment of the depth compensation control for the correct recording of the interventricular septum

amplitude of about 10 mm for about 0,36 sec[5] [50]. This motion is preceded by a small posterior movement (atrial contraction). At the end of systole it has a rapid posterior motion (lasting 0,08 to 0,10 sec) during rapid early diastolic filling; during the slow left ventricular filling phase, slight posterior motion is observed. The diastolic thickness of the posterior wall is measured from the most anterior endocardial echo to the most anterior epicardial echo; it is usually the same thickness as the interventricular septum[43] [189] [206]. The systolic thickness is measured at its maximal thickness[42].

M mode scanning towards the apex explores other regions of the ventricle (distal 1/3 of the septum and the posterior wall), as the internal dimension of the cavity progressively decreases. The amplitude of wall motion is exaggerated by the obliquity of the ultrasonic beam[54]. Sometimes, it is possible to record part of the postero-medial papillary muscle anterior to the posterior wall.

The apical part of the anterior wall may be recorded in some patients by gliding the transducer laterally over the chest wall[33].

The LV may also be studied by the same method from the subcostal position: the LV internal dimension so obtained is another short axis which, in practice, is of the same size as that measured from the left parasternal position[194]. However, it is the inferior portion of the interventricular septum and the lateral wall of the left ventricle which are visualised.

3.2.3. Study of the left ventricular performance

The ability to record the left ventricle in diastole and systole provides a means of evaluating left ventricular performance[119] [141].

Although M mode echo only gives a unidimensional view, it does give good definition of the left ventricular walls and their motion throughout the cardiac cycle: 2D studies give a global appreciation of the geometry of the cavity, but the definition of the endocardium is not as good. This is a source of error in the measurement of the left ventricular dimensions by this method.

In practice, M mode studies remain valuable in the assessment of the quality of myocardial contractility.

A) M mode

• **Ventricular volumes:** (fig. 3-51)

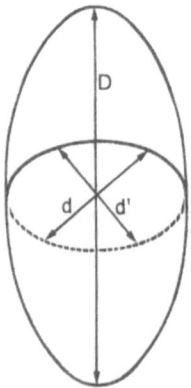

Fig. 3-51 The left ventricle may be compared to a prolate ellipse, the two short axes (d and d') being equal, and the long axis (D) being twice the short axis:

$$(d = d' = \frac{D}{2})$$

Assuming that the left ventricle may be described as a prolate ellipse with a long axis twice the length of its short axes (fig. 3-51), and knowing the value (d) of one of the short axes, it becomes possible to calculate the ventricular volume by the following formula[51]:

$$V = \frac{4}{3} \times \pi \times \frac{D}{2} \times \frac{d'}{2} \times \frac{d}{2}$$

$$V = volume$$

$$but \ d = d' = D/2$$

$$Therefore \ V = \frac{4}{3} \pi \times \frac{d^3}{4} \simeq d^3$$

According to this formula, the enddiastolic volume equals the cube of the enddiastolic internal dimension and the endsystolic volume equals the cube of the systolic internal dimension[54] [159bis]. Any error in the measurement of the internal dimension will be cubed in the estimation of the volumes[125].

As the ventricle dilates, its form becomes more spherical and the values of the long and short axes approximate each other. Several correction factors have been suggested to compensate for this distortion[59] [107] [203] ; Teicholz's formula[203] seems to be the most satisfactory one[107] giving the best correlations with dilution and angiographic methods of measuring ventricular volume.

$$V = \frac{7}{2,4 + d} \times d^3$$

For ventricles with normal enddiastolic internal dimensions (d = 4,6 cm) this correction factor is not required and the cube formula V = d³ may be used. These methods seem to be reliable for the calculation of diastolic volumes (Vd) in all pathologies. However, in coronary heart disease, the calculation of the systolic volume (Vs) is erroneous as segmental abnormalities of myocardial contraction are not allowed for[202] [203].

Bearing these limitations in mind, stroke volume (SV) may be calculated by the following formula:

$$SV = Vd - Vs$$

and the cardiac output by multiplying SV by the heart rate.

• **Left ventricular mass** (LV mass)

The calculation of LV mass depends upon echocardiographic measurement of volumes; the internal diastolic volume is subtracted from the volume of the ventricle including the thickness of its two walls, and the whole is multiplied by 1,05, the specific gravity of cardiac muscle[206].

$$\text{LV mass} = [(\text{LVIDd} + \text{PWT} + \text{SWT})^3 - \text{LVIDd}^3] \times 1,05$$

LVIDd = diastolic LV dimension
WT = diastolic posterior wall thickness
SWT = diastolic septal thickness
LV mass = ventricular mass in grammes if the dimensions are in centimetres

LV mass may also be obtained with Teicholz's correction.

In practice, these results are expressed as the LV mass index:
LV mass in grammes/m² body surface area
normal = 97 ± 23 g/m²

• **Ejection fraction** (EF)

This is estimated by the same method as used in angiography.

$$\text{EF} = \frac{\text{Vd} - \text{Vs}}{\text{Vd}} \times 100 = \frac{\text{SV}}{\text{VD}} \times 100$$

These results are subject to the same errors as the calculation of volumes. The normal value is 72 %, which is higher than that obtained by angiographic methods. This is due to the fact that the EF is only calculated with respect to circumferential shortening which is greater than the shortening of the long axis[44] which is taken into consideration in the angiographic method.

• **Peripheral vascular resistance**[195] (R)

It is possible to calculate with simultaneous echocardiographic recording and blood pressure measurement:

$$R = \frac{\text{Mean Arterial Pressure}}{\text{Cardiac Output}}$$

- Factional shortening of the left ventricle

To eliminate inherent errors in volume measurement, the calculation of the fractional shortening of the left ventricle has been suggested as an equivalent of the ejection fraction[54][109].

$$\% \text{ shortening} = \frac{\text{LVIDd} - \text{LVIDs}}{\text{LIVDd}} \times 100$$

This index of left ventricular performance has become widely used for several reasons: it is independant of age and heart rate, it is less subject to observer error and its easy to calculate. The average normal value is 36 %. It constitutes an easy method of detecting impaired ventricular performance and is very useful in following-up patients.

- Mean rate of circumferential fiber shortening (mean VCF)[32][60][152]:

This index requires measurement of the left ventricular ejection time. This may be estimated by measuring the contraction time (CT) of the left ventricular posterior wall from the onset of QRS to the point of maximal thickness and subtracting 0.05 sec to allow for the isovolumic contraction time. LV ejection time may be more reliably measured either directly from the aortic valves (opening to closure, although this is usually not simultaneous) or from simultaneous external carotid pulse recordings.

$$\text{mean VCF} = \frac{\text{LVIDd} - \text{LVIDs}}{\text{LVIDd} \times \text{ET}}$$

$$(\text{normal} = 1,18 \text{ circumferences/sec.})$$

This index varies with heart rate[38], age[81], preload and afterload[93]. Despite these limits it remains a sensitive index of ventricular performance.

- Analysis of wall thickening:

The systolic thickening of the left ventricular walls visualised on M mode investigation may be analysed:

— *Percentage thickening: % T*

$$\% \text{ T} = \frac{\text{Ts} - \text{Td}}{\text{Td}} \times 100$$

Ts = systolic thickness
Td = diastolic thickness

normal = 62% (for the LV posterior wall).

$$\frac{V.Tw}{C} = \frac{Ts - Td}{Td \times CT}$$

Normal $= 1{,}75 \ \mu Tw/s$ (for the LV posterior wall).

Where CT is the contraction time of the wall under study. Septal contraction time is usually shorter than posterior wall contraction time.

These indices of thickening are normally lower for the septum. They reflect the integrity of regional contraction[42][43][44]: standard scanning towards the apex allows study of serial segments. When these views are combined with recordings of the anterior and lateral walls (from the subcostal position), a qualitative and quantitative assessment of regional contractility becomes possible in all these areas. Reduction of these indices implies "hypokinetic" wall motion, absence of wall thickening "akinesia", and systolic thinning is a sign of "dyskinesia"[42] (see chapter on Coronary Heart Disease).

● Assessment of hypertrophy

The $\frac{h}{r}$ ratio (h = diastolic wall thickness; r = internal diastolic radius) is normally 0.36. Its value increases slightly with age[166]. This ratio has been suggested as a means of identifying excentric hypertrophy when it is normal[80] from concentric hypertrophy (increased ratio)[43][64].

● Computer assisted analysis of left ventricular performance:

Echocardiographic information can be entered into a computer by manually tracing the echos with a position sensitive graph pen. All the previously described indices may be calculated instantaneously and a number of successive cycles analysed.

The instantaneous rates of change of diameter and thickening, measurements which are impossible manually, may be easily obtained[156][204][210].

Recent publications have shown the value and sensitivity of computer assisted analysis of echocardiographic data, especially in the study of left ventricular filling.

Other advantages are the possibility of stocking the information for research studies and the computerised printout of results.

B) *2D* : 2D echo evaluation of left ventricular performance is not yet routine practice; it is, at present, under validation both on experimental models and by comparison with other techniques. 2D echo offsets the approximations used in M mode. 2D sections in different, preferably perpendicular planes, allow the calculation of the volume at each moment of the cardiac cycle by the same formulae as are used in angiography; however, the sections are not simultaneous and so usually only the end-diastolic and endsystolic volumes are calculated[66].

The correlation with angiography is good, with a slight tendency to underestimate the volumes with 2D[21] [58] [179] echo; the angiographic view corresponds to the projection of left ventricular volume in one plane and therefore higher values are obtained. In 2D examination, the largest dimension is not automatically obtained in each section. Depite these differences, the correlations for the calculation of the ejection fractions are very good[21] [58]. The left ventricular mass may also be calculated in the same way. Recent studies suggest that it may soon be possible to reconstitute an image of the left ventricle in movement in three dimensions: sequential transverse sections are positioned in space and stored in a computer which, after integrating all the information, would reconstitute an image of the left ventricle in the desired incidence[46] [207].

The method described above would visualise the ventricular walls, and theoretically allow a segmental analysis of regional wall movement. However, this would be essentially a qualitative assessment as the myocardium is not always sufficiently well defined with 2D echo for assessment of wall thickening[162].

The use of simultaneous M mode echo would make precise quantitative analysis of regional wall function possible. 2D scanning would be used to localise the anatomical zone under study and M mode would make available the indices of wall thickening in all zone explored.

PART II:

CONGENITAL HEART DISEASE

The recording of an echocardiogram in children, infants or premature babies is often difficult[191]; the child must be calm (sometimes, mild sedation is required) and warm (examination of babies in an incubator), and a great deal of operator skill and wide knowledge of congenital heart disease are necessary. The investigation should be performed and interpreted with respect to the clinical context in order to guide the choice of complementary investigations and therapy, especially in neonatal emergencies: when faced with the problem of cardiac failure, echo can distinguish between cardiomyopathy, hypoplasia of one cavity and a shunt.

Transducers of higher frequency (3,5 to 7 MHz) are used, giving better proximal, axial and lateral resolution.

2D echo gives information on the spatial orientation of the malformations whilst M-mode gives an appreciation of their physiopathological repercussions.

Ultrasound contrast techniques may be used to outline blood flow to detect intracardiac shunts. In practice, this procedure requires an intravenous injection in the forearm, or the umbilical vein in neonates[182].

CHAPTER 4

RIGHT HEART MALFORMATIONS

4.1. RIGHT VENTRICULAR DIASTOLIC OVERLOAD

These conditions are characterised by increased right ventricular volume [39] [197] and RV/LV ratio [118]. Systolic septal motion is often paradoxical (fig. 4-1, 4-2), especially in severe cases, due to inversion of the septal curvature by the volume overload, so that during systole, the septum moves anteriorly towards the RV, when the transducer is positoned in the parasternal area (fig. 4-3, 4-4).

Although this movement is abnormal, septal contraction is effective as normal systolic thickening is observed [65] (fig.4-2).

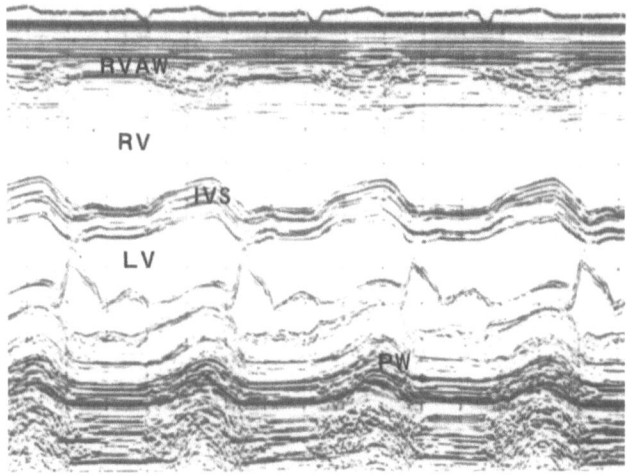

Fig. 4-1

M mode recording showing right ventricular diastolic overload and type A paradoxical septal motion

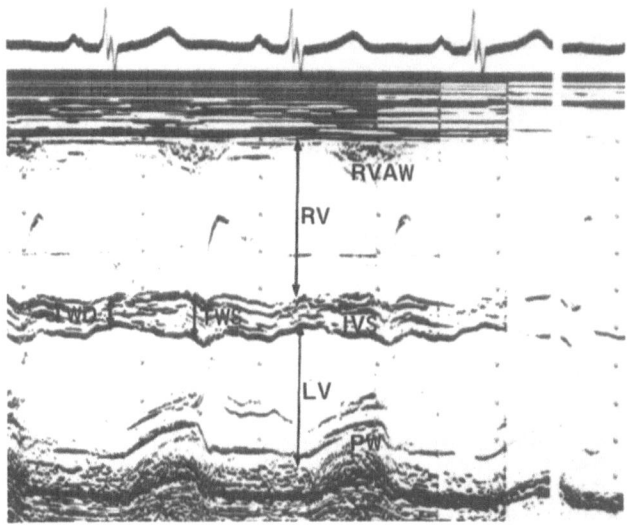

Fig. 4-2

M mode recording showing right ventricular diastolic overload and type B paradoxical septal motion. There is a significant increase in the RV/ LV ratio (> 1)

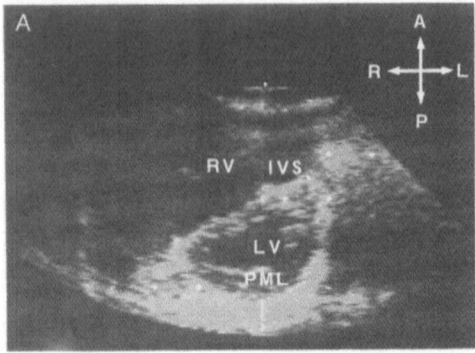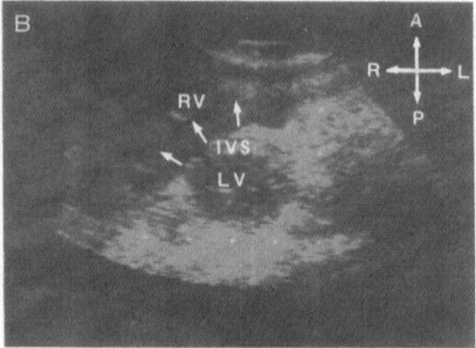

*Fig. 4-3 Right ventricular diastolic overload 2D short axis views
   A- Diastolic frame: Septal curvature is inverted. The left ventricle appears to
   be smaller than the dilated right ventricle
   B- Systolic frame: the interventricular septum contracts towards the right
   ventricle

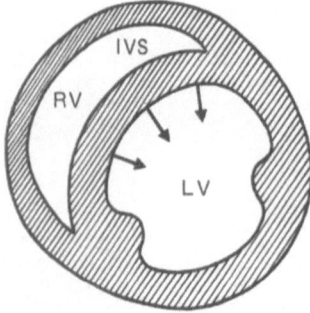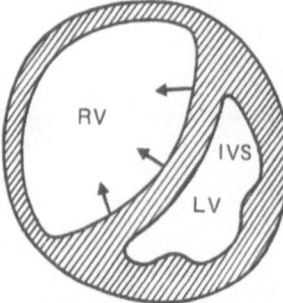

Fig. 4-4 A- Normal septal position
at the end of diastole. In systole
the septum contracts towards the
left ventricular posterior wall and
posterior motion is recorded on
M mode
   B- In right ventricular
diastolic overload, the diastolic
curvature of the septum is inverted.
In systole, it contracts towards
the right ventricle giving an
anterior septal motion on M mode

A- Normal   B- Right ventricular diastolic overload

Paradoxical septal motion is not specific for right ventricular volume overload. It may be recorded after open heart surgery or in congenital absence of the pericardium[15] [154], pulmonary embolism[101] [120bis], restrictive syndromes of the right heart[69], conduction defects[129], etc.

4.1.1. Atrial septal defect (ASD)

A) *Anatomy:* this malformation is caused by incomplete septation of the atria and results in a left-right shunt.

The following forms may be distinguished :

- ostium secundum involving the mid part of the septum (the most common)

- sinus venosus (the rarest) located in the dorsal part of the septum

- ostium primum defects involving the septum in its continuity with the atrioventricular valves; according to the severity of the lesion, the valves and the interventricular septum may be affected so realising complete or incomplete forms of endocardial cushion defect (see further on).

Other malformations are frequently associated with ASD:

partial anomalous pulmonary venous return (very common in sinus venosus), mitral valve prolapse (one third of secundum defects), pulmonary stenosis. ASD may also form an integral part of a more complex cardiac malformation.

B) *Diagnostic signs:* besides the common signs of right ventricular diastolic overload, atrial septal defect and its location may be directly visualised by 2D echo. The best incidence for studying the interatrial septum is when the ultrasound beam is perpendicular, that is to say the subcostal long axis view[10] (fig. 4-5).

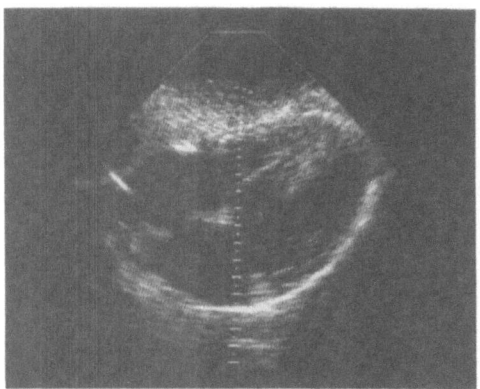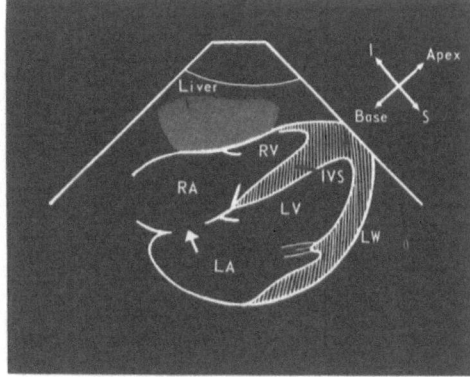

Fig. 4-5 2D subcostal view: direct visualization of an ostium secundum atrial septal defect

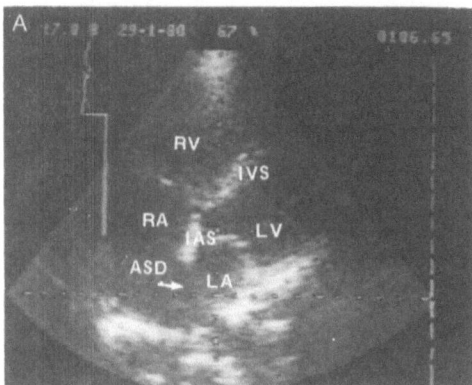

Fig. 4-6

2D apical view: contrast study in a patient with atrial septal defect. The arrow indicates the negative image due to the left-to-right atrial shunt

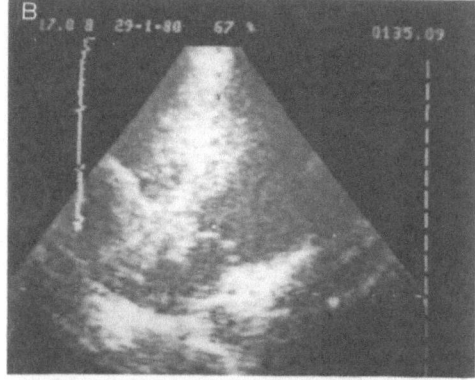

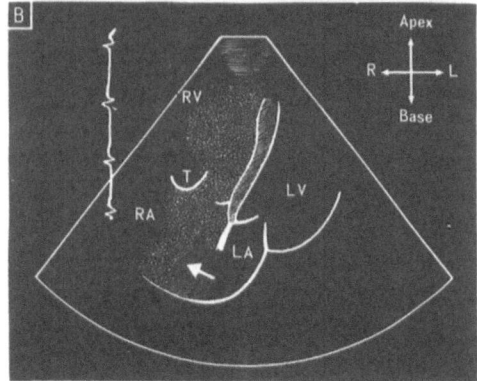

The left-right shunt may be demonstrated by ''negative'' contrast images in the right atrium whilst right-left shunts give rise to opacification of the left atrium (fig. 4-6)[61] [233](fig. 4-6 bis).

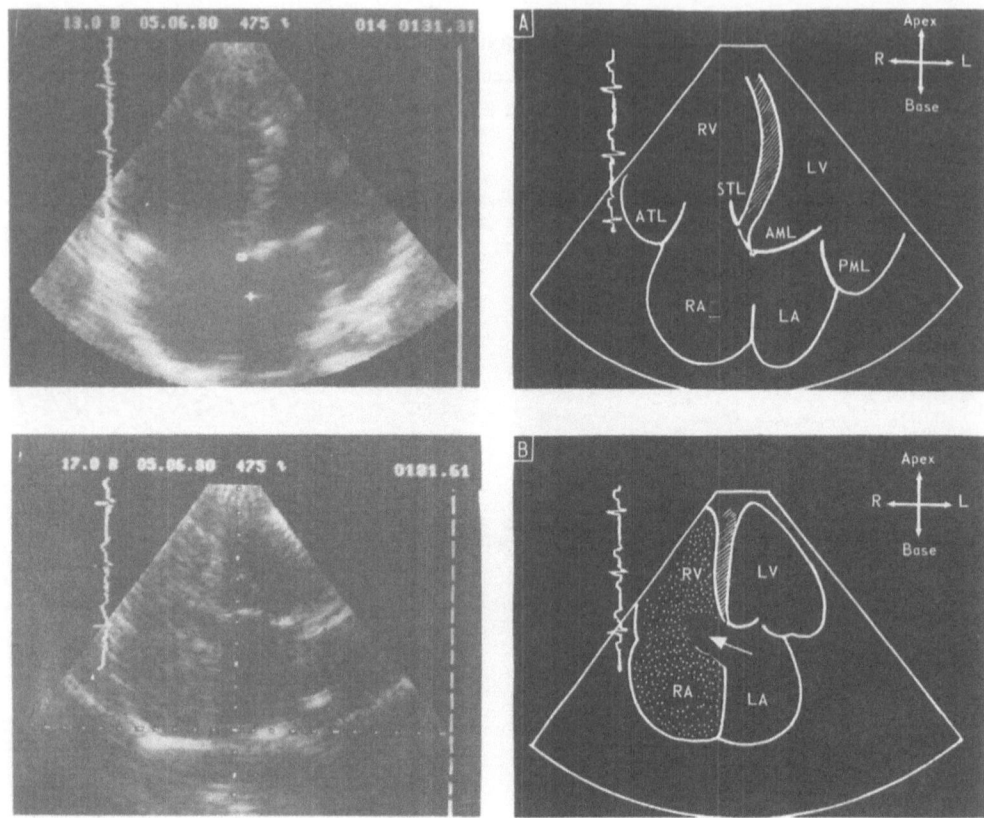

Fig. 4-6 bis Ostium primum ASD
A- Apical view: diastolic frame. The RV is dilated and the interventricular septum bulges into the LV. The borders of the ASD are marked with asterisks
B- Contrast: The negative jet is arrowed

The septal defect cannot be visualised on M-mode, but the association of mitral valve prolapse is suggestive of an ostium secundum (ASD)[9] and abnormalities of the left ventricular outflow tract, an ostium primum ASD (fig. 4-7) (mitral regurgitation, cleft mitral valve, corresponding to the typical ''goose neck'' appearance on angiography)[236] (fig. 4-8). An assessment of the size of the shunt may be obtained on M-mode by calculating the RV/LV ratio. A normal RV/LV ratio excludes a significant left-right shunt at atrial level[118]. The pulmonary valve is usually easy to record (pulmonary artery dilatation); premature opening suggests associated pulmonary stenosis[223], but a large A wave is often recorded in ASDs with large shunts in the absence of any pulmonary valvular lesion (fig. 4-9). The absence of an A wave and midsystolic closure is suggestive of pulmonary hypertension[224].

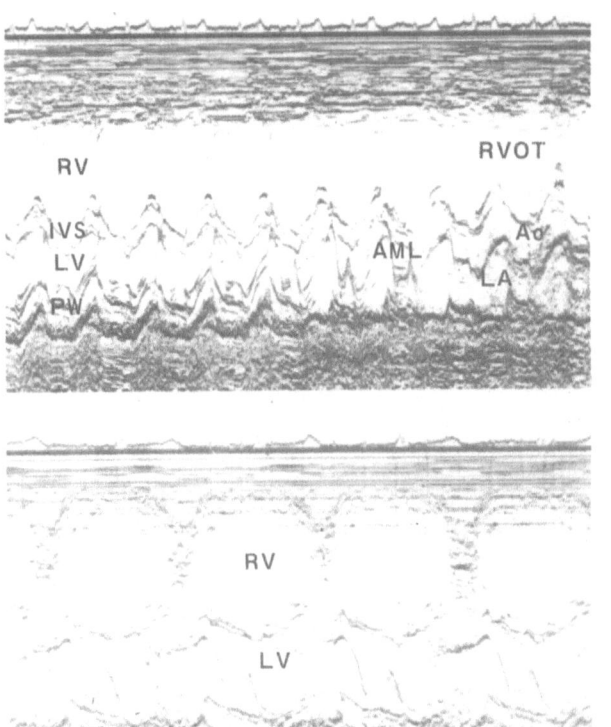

Fig. 4-7
M mode recordings of ostium primum atrial septal defect. The abnormality of the systolic portion of the mitral valve in the left ventricular outflow tract is shown (arrow)

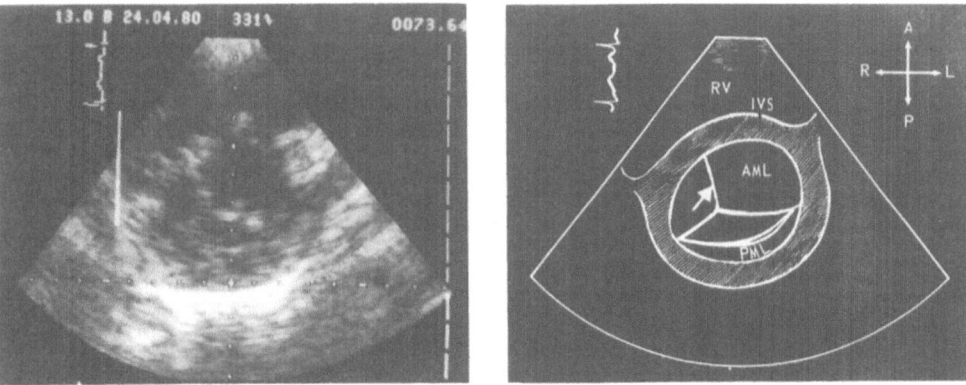

Fig. 4-8 2D short axis view in ostium primum atrial septal defect. This systolic frame shows the cleft anterior mitral leaflet responsible for mitral regurgitation

The tricuspid valve is usually visualised very well because of right ventricular dilatation. It has a large amplitude of opening (due to increased blood flow) with respect to the mitral valve, and sometimes fine diastolic fluttering may be recorded (large shunts)[144] (fig. 4-9). The left ventricular internal dimensions may be reduced but the indices of left ventricular function remain within normal limits[37].

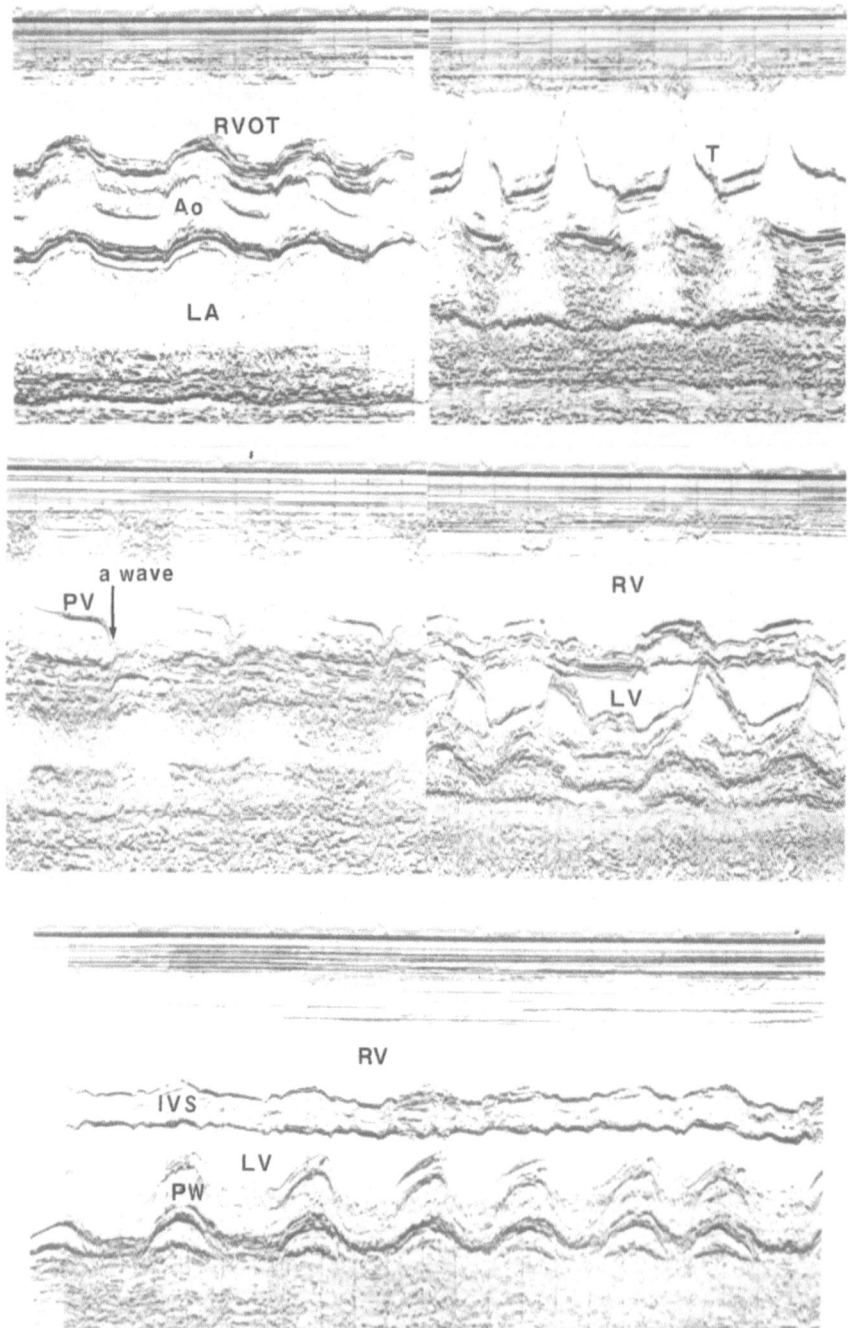

Fig. 4-9 M mode recording of the four cardiac valves in ostium secundum atrial septal defect. TV: tricuspid valve wich is unusually well recorded because of right ventricular dilatation PV: pulmonary valve showing a deep "a" wave, suggestive of a large left-to-right shunt

Reliable measurement of the right ventricular internal dimension requires good quality recordings of the right ventricular anterior wall and the right border of the septum. This necessitates correct adjustement of the time gain compensation and adaptation of the depth of examination to the size of the heart in order to avoid reverberations which may falsify the measurements (fig. 1-8).

Recording is performed in the supine position as the right ventricular internal dimension is increased by turning the patient on his left side[54], and lead to a false positive diagnosis of ASD.

The interventricular septum is studied in the routine ventricular incidence. It is only at this level that one can diagnose paradoxical motion as the subaortic interventricular septum normally moves anteriorly in systole (transmitted aortic motion)[86].

With 2D echo a false image of atrial septal defect may be observed in the area of the fossa ovalis in apical views[188]. Direct visualisation of ASD can only be confirmed with subcostal views[10].

Partial abnormal pulmonary venous return (APVR) cannot be visualised by M-mode and gives rise to the same signs of right ventricular diastolic overload[237]. They may sometimes be seen directly with 2D or indirectly with contrast techniques (see further on).

Other causes of right ventricular diastolic overload usually have specific clinical and echocardiographic diagnostic criteria. However, it is difficult to distinguish between adult forms of ASD with pulmonary hypertension from severe pulmonary hypertension due to other causes; in these circumstances, the diagnosis of primary ASD or patent foramen ovale can only be made by opacification of the LA by echocardiographic contrast techniques[61].

Immediate and long-term postoperative echocardiography should be part of routine follow-up of patients operated for ASD.

• The patch may be visualised with 2D echo[188].

• The RV/LV ratio decreases very rapidly and should return to normal about twelve months after surgery: in the absence of severe preoperative pulmonary hypertension, persistance of the echocardiographic signs of right ventricular overload suggests a residual shunt (patch failure, uncorrected partial APVR, uncorrected multiple ASD). Septal motion follows the evolution of the RV/LV ratio[118].

4.1.2. Endocardial cushion defect (ECD)

A) *Anatomy*[142]:

ECD is caused by incomplete development of the endocardial cushions.
This results in variable anomalies of the lower part of the interatrial septum, the atrioventricular valves and the upper part of the interventricular septum, giving rise to partial or complete forms of atrioventricular canal.

The most common manifestations are ostium primum ASD, a ventricular septal defect

(VSD) and abnormal insertion of the atrioventricular valves, both located lower down in the ventricle and in the same plane. One (complete type) or two valvular rings (partial type) may be present with common or separate papillary muscles. The echocardiographic findings will depend on the type of anatomical abnormality which is present and vary from ostium primum ASD to an extreme form of single ventricle with only one atrioventricular valve.

ECDs are often isolated abnormalities but an association with Fallot's tetralogy, corrected transposition of the great vessels, asplenia, may be encountered.

B) *Diagnostic signs :*

M-mode : the recording of an echo of an atrioventricular valve apparently transversing the interventricular septal echo is considered to be the best sign of a common valve in complete forms of ECD[236]. However, this has also been described in partial forms of the anomaly[82] where careful scanning is required to demonstrate the two atrioventricular valves simultaneously without intervening septal echo (fig. 4-10). As in ostium primum ASD, the mitral valve is situated more anteriorly and there is narrowing of the left ventricular outflow tract.

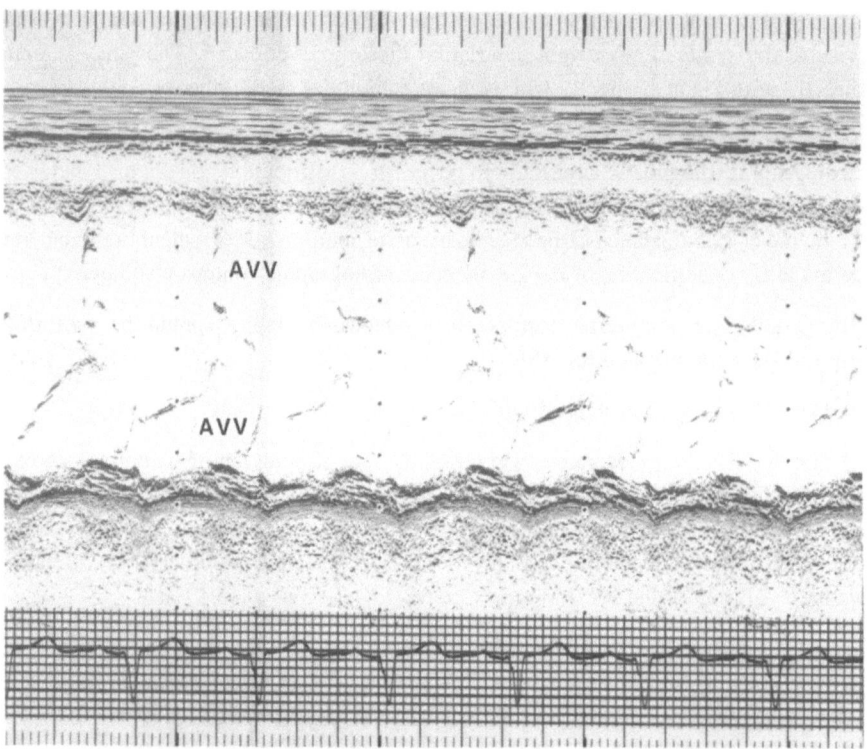

Fig. 4-10 M mode echocardiogram of a severe endocardial cushion defect with a large ventricular septal defect: there appear to be two atrioventricular valves. Scanning down towards the apex confirmed the presence of an interventricular septum, so excluding the diagnosis of single ventricle

AVV: atrioventricular valve

In complete forms of ECD the interventricular septum is not visualised at the base of the heart. In the routine ventricular incidence, normal septal motion is recorded despite right ventricular dilatation[237]; left ventricular volume overload is also present, causing dilatation of the left heart cavities[134].

The anatomical lesion may be visualised by 2D echo with helps in the interpretation of the M-mode scans. The size of the VSD, the presence of one or both atrioventricular valves, details of the insertion of their chordae are essential pieces of information for the surgeon[84] (fig. 4-11)(fig. 4-11bis).

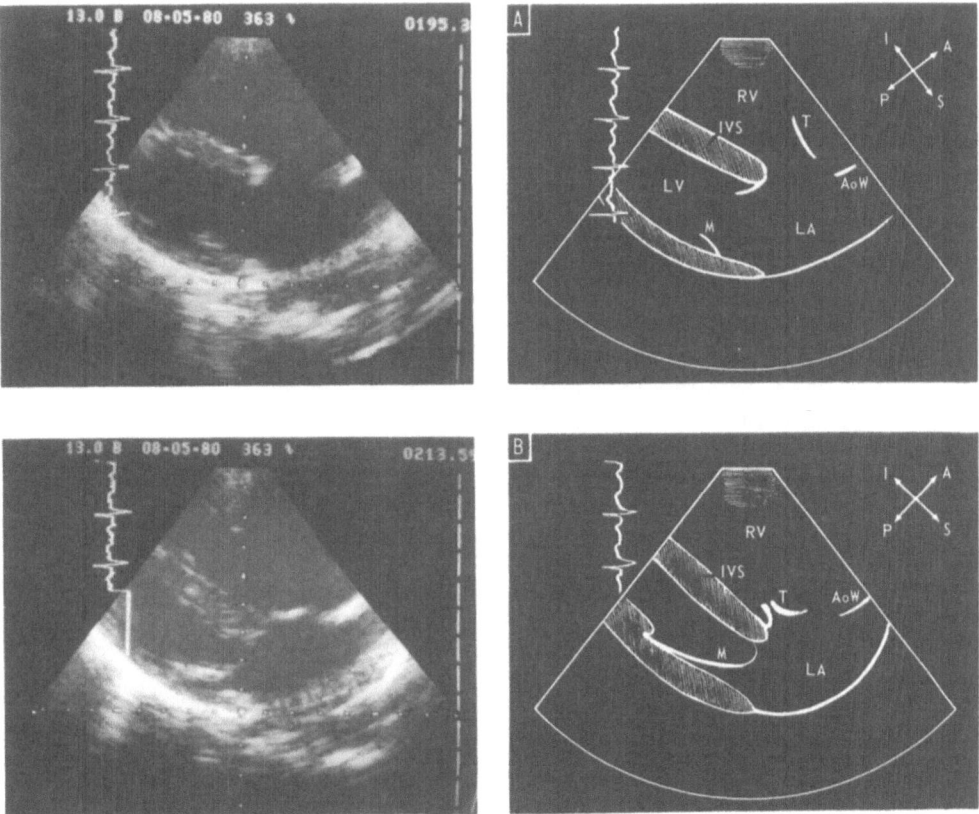

Fig. 4-11 A partial form of endocardial cushion defect
A- 2D long axis view: diastolic frame showing the ventricular septal defect and two atrioventricular valves
B- The same view: systolic frame

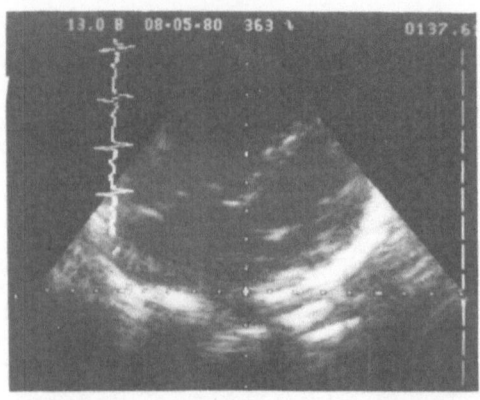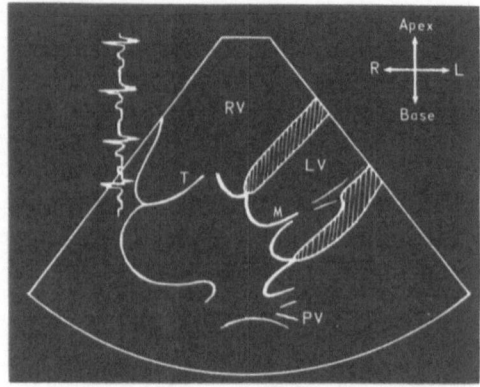

Fig. 4·11 bis Endocardial cushion defect apical 4 chamber view.
The two atrioventricular valves and a large ASD are visualised

The presence, level and relative size of right-left shunts can be studied by contrast echocardiography (fig. 4-12).

C) *Diagnostic pitfalls and comments:*

The complexity of the various forms of ECD make M-mode echo difficult to interpret: repeated scanning is necessary to show the interventricular septum and the presence of two valves in separate cavities[154].

The main differential diagnosis is that of single ventricle which may have the same presentation of a single atrioventricular valve and absence of the interventricular septum. However, the vestigial anterior chamber may be visualised by 2D echo (see chapter 7).

One diagnosis that must be excluded is that of overriding tricuspid valve (see chapter 7).

Finally, in single atrium, signs of a partial form of ECD are recorded but 2D echo shows the absence of an interatrial septum[185].

Fig. 4·12 A- M mode left-to-right scan in the same patient as in fig. 4-11, showing the mitral, the tricuspid and then both valves together, the latter seeming to traverse the interventricular septum
B- Contrast study on a simultaneous M mode recording: contrast appears behind the mitral valve suggesting a right-to-left shunt at atrial level

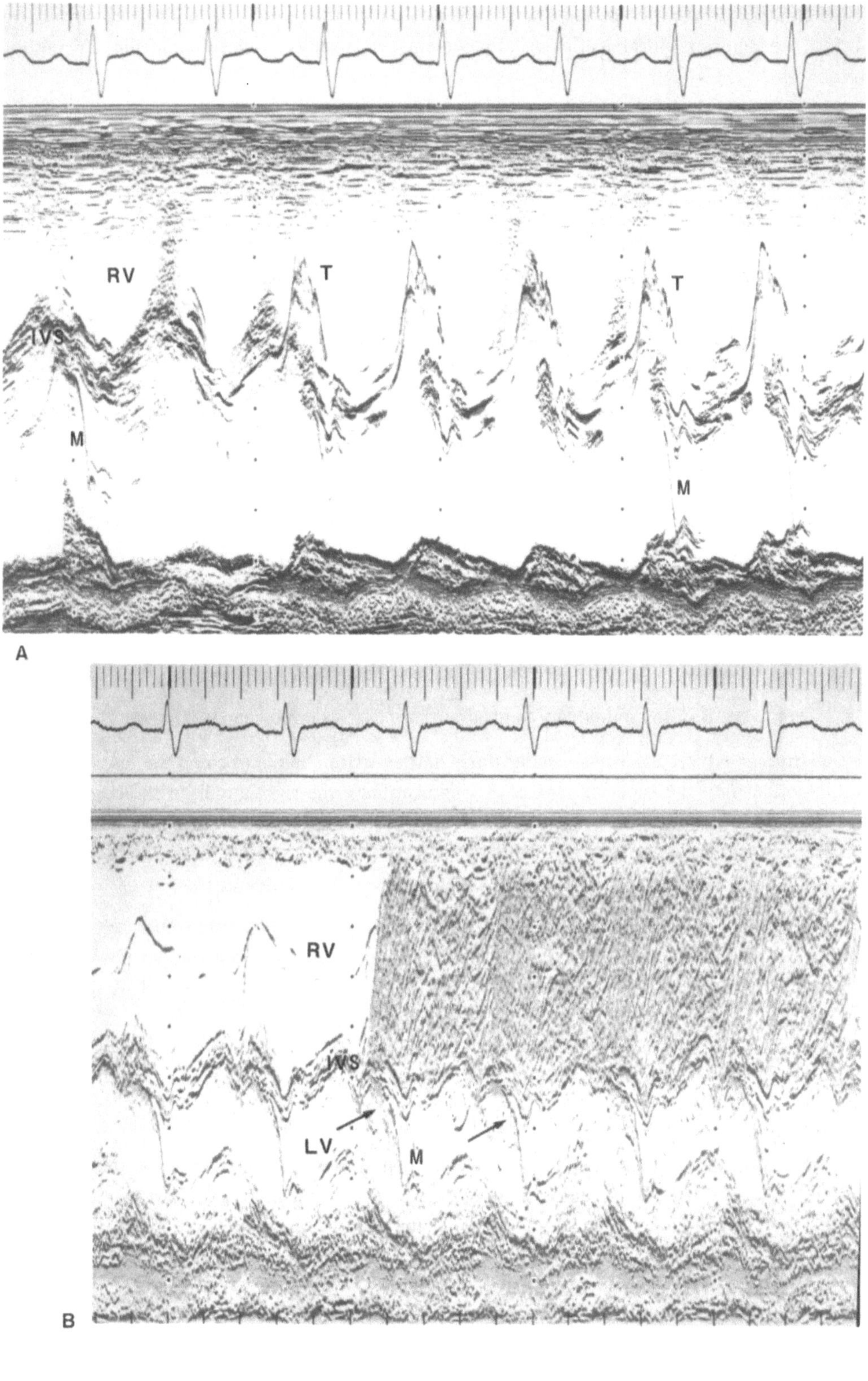

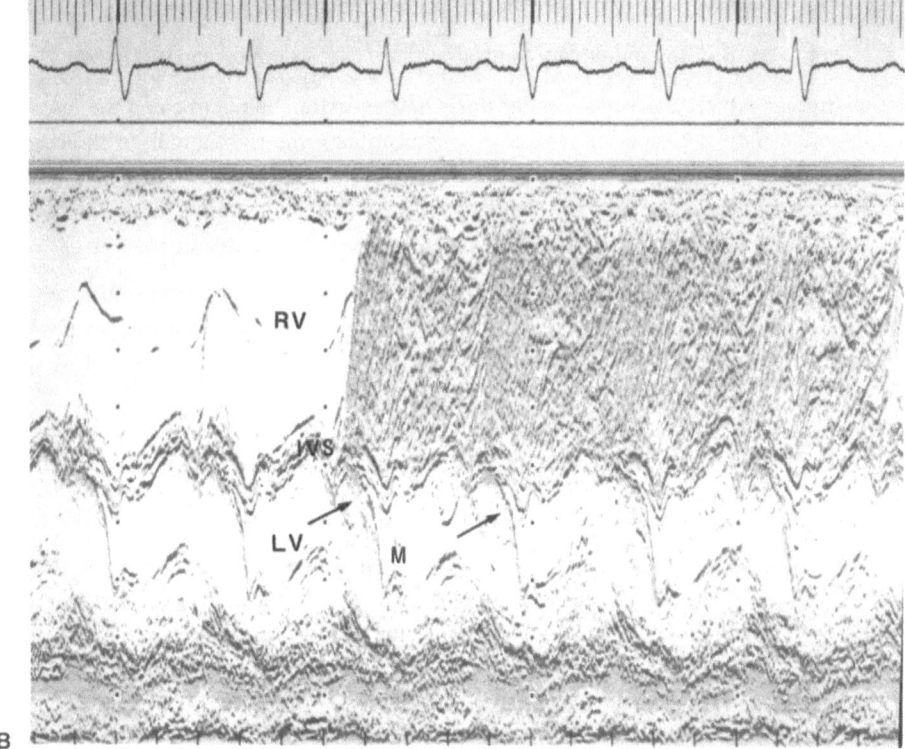

A

B

In the postoperative period the patch is easily recorded, especially with apical views (fig. 4-13): the anterior mitral leaflet usually remains in an anterior position in the LV outflow tract[237].

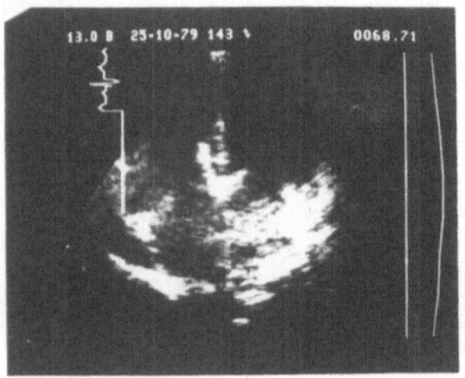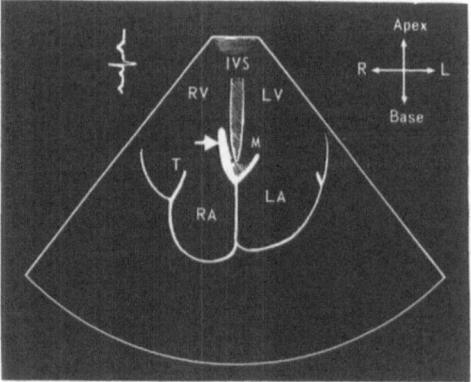

Fig. 4-13 2D 4 chamber view: endocardial cushion defect after correction. The patch on the right septal border is marked with an arrow

4.1.3. Anomalous pulmonary venous return (APVR)

A) *Anatomy:*

Some or all of the pulmonary veins drain into the systemic venous circulation.

In total APVR the veins usually drain into an extra chamber behind the LA which itself drains either into the superior vena cava (supracardiac), the right atrium or the coronary sinus (intracardiac), the inferior vena cava (infracardiac)[31]. This abnormality is a neonatal emergency and survival is only possible when ASD or patent foramen ovale are present. In 1/3 cases, another congenital malformation is associated.

In partial left APVR, the left pulmonary veins also drain into a chamber behind the LA, but in the right pulmonary forms, the veins drain directly into the systemic venous circulation. An ASD is very commonly associated[142].

B) *Diagnostic signs:*

In all cases, the same signs of right ventricular diastolic overload are recorded.

• Total APVR

M-mode: Paquet and Gutgesell[151] were the first workers to describe the presence of an echo-free space behind the LA corresponding to the common pulmonary venous chamber which was identified by contrast technique during retrograde catheterisation (fig. 4-14, 4-15).

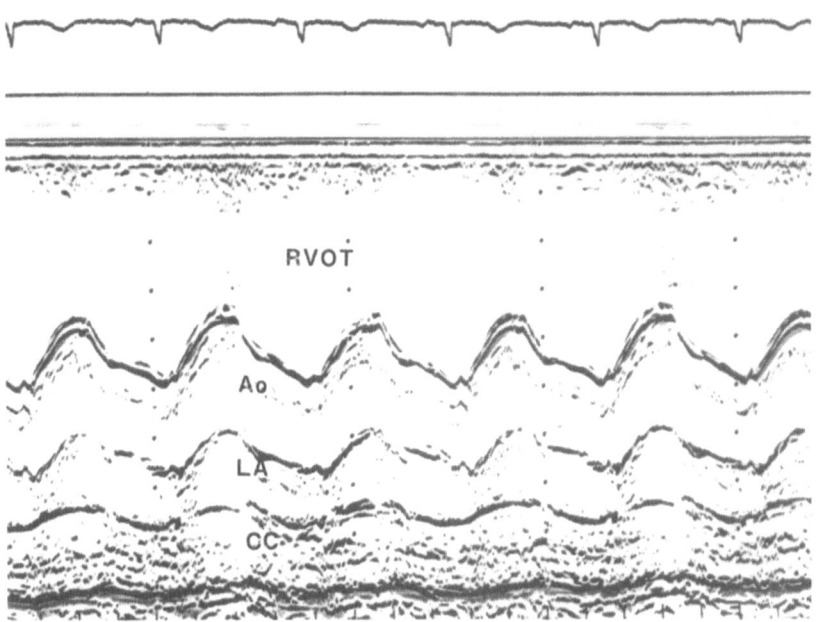

Fig. 4-14 Left atrial echogramm showing the common pulmonary venous chamber (CC) in a case of total anomalous pulmonary venous return   CC: common chamber

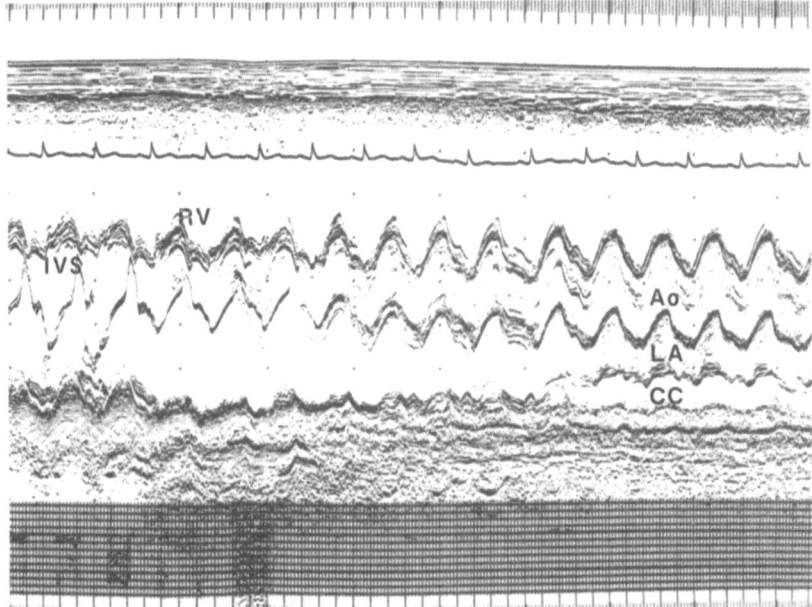

Fig. 4-15 Total anomalous pulmonary venous return. M mode scan showing the common pulmonary venous chamber (CC) behind the left atrium (LA) and right ventricular diastolic overload

2D: the common pulmonary venous chamber is directly visualised in parasternal and apical ong axis views (fig. 4-16). Sahn et al. have recently shown that it is possible to study the drainage of the pulmonary veins, diagnose and distinguish the forms of TAPVR[175] (see fig. 3-38).

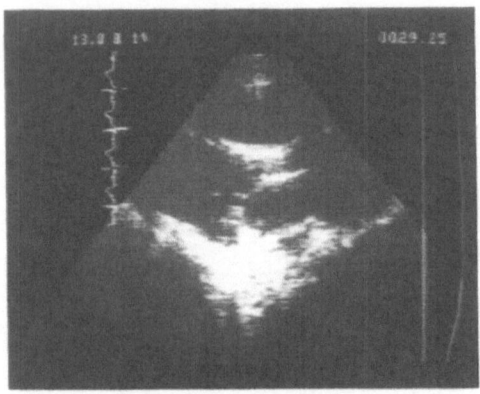 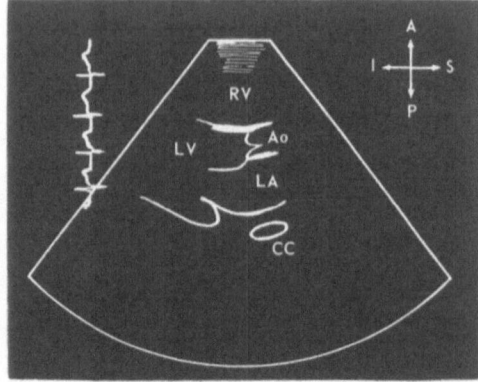

Fig. 4-16 2D long axis view: total anomalous pulmonary venous return. The oval, echo-free space behind the left atrium (LA) corresponds to the common pulmonary venous chamber (CC). Note the right ventricular dilatation (RV)

When total APVR drains into the coronary sinus, its dilatation may be visualised both by M-mode and 2D echo as a circular echo free space at the left atrioventricular junction; the common pulmonary venous chamber is situated in a much more posterior position behind the LA[150].

The presence of a small left ventricular cavity has been described as a poor prognostic sign in the post operative course after complete correction[237].

● **Partial APVR**

Only partial left APVR drains into a common chamber behind the LA. The echocardiographic signs of an echo free space behind the LA are identical to those of total APVR, but the clinical situation is not urgent and the signs of right ventricular overload are not as severe.

Partial right APVR gives rise to signs of right ventricular diastolic overload. In the absence of ASD, certain negative signs such as the integrity of the interatrial septum and the absence of a negative jet in the right atrium during contrast techniques may suggest the diagnosis.

C) *Diagnostic pitfalls and comments:*

All forms of APVR pose the same technical and diagnostic problems as other malformations giving rise to right ventricular diastolic overload. More specifically, to confirm the presence of a common pulmonary venous chamber, other causes of an echo free space in the left atrial region must be excluded:

● a large pericardial effusion may extend behind the LA, but this echo free space is in continuity with the classical appearances of pericardial effusion behind the ventricle (see Tome II).

● the descending thoracic aorta: this structure is commonly recorded normally as a circular echo free space, the position of which varies depending on whether it is recorded on a longitudinal or transverse view[139] (fig. 4-17). However, it is clearly retrocardiac and may be unfolded and seen to be continuous with careful scanning (see fig. 3-11).

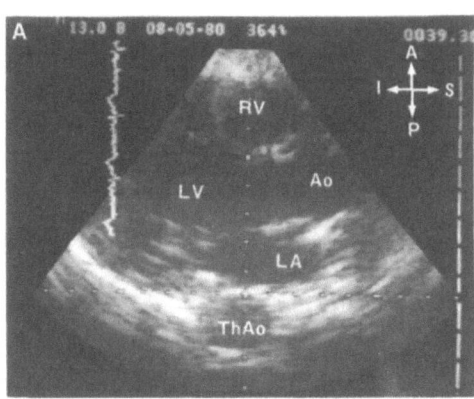

Fig. 4-17

Echogram·of the descending thoracic aorta (ThAo)
  A- 2D long axis view showing the descending thoracic aorta as a circular retrocardiac echo-free space

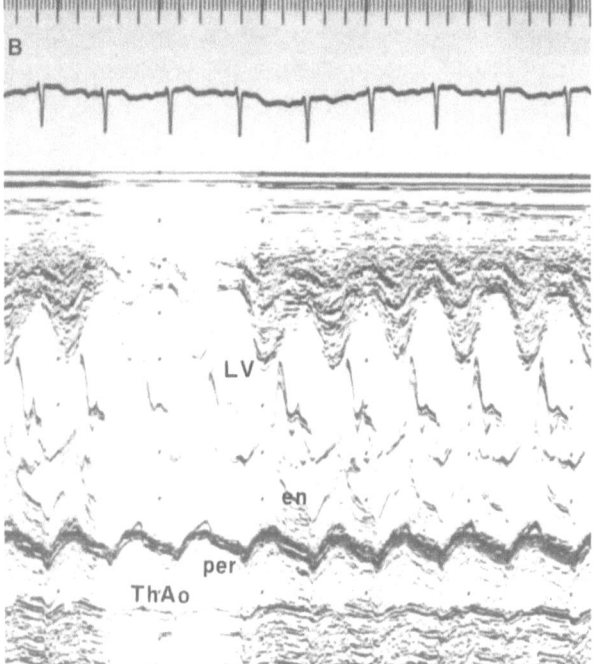

B- M mode recording showing the thoracic aorta as on echo-free space behind the left ventricular posterior wall

● dilatation of the coronary sinus: besides APVR to the coronary sinus, the coronary sinus may also be dilated in cases of abnormal systemic venous return due to persistent left superior vena cava (fig. 4-18).

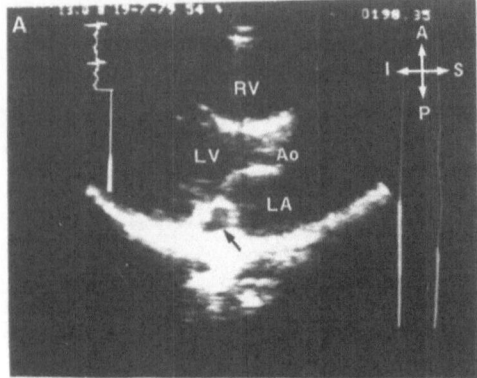

Fig. 4-18

A- 2D long axis view showing dilatation of the coronary sinus (left superior vena cava and anomalous systemic venous return to the coronary sinus) situated at the atrioventricular junction

B- Simultaneous M mode showing the coronary sinus (CS) at the atrioventricular junction

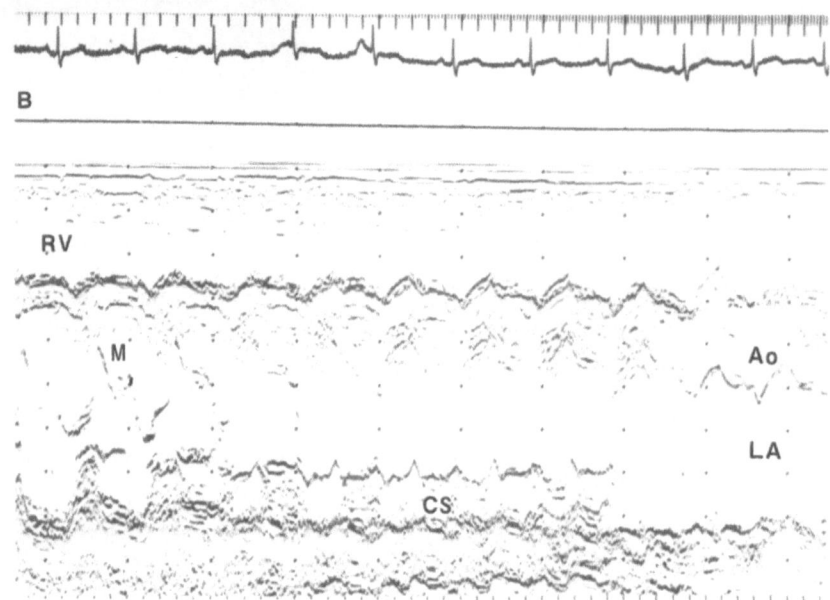

The diagnosis is made by contrast technique; injection into a left arm vein results in opacification of the coronary sinus followed by the right heart cavities[190] (fig. 4-19).

• cor triatriatum: in this abnormality the abnormal echo is intraatrial, but the differential diagnosis of a common pulmonary venous chamber is extremely difficult by both M-mode and 2D echo, especially when there is an associated ASD[19]. In the new born, the clinical and echocardiographic signs are similar. In our experience, the various forms of APVR may be diagnosed correctly with a combination of 2D and M-mode echo, but the non-visualisation of the common pulmonary venous chamber does not exclude the diagnosis.

The pulmonary venous chamber may be visualised post operatively and a persistent increased RV/LV ratio is recorded when ASD is left unrepaired.

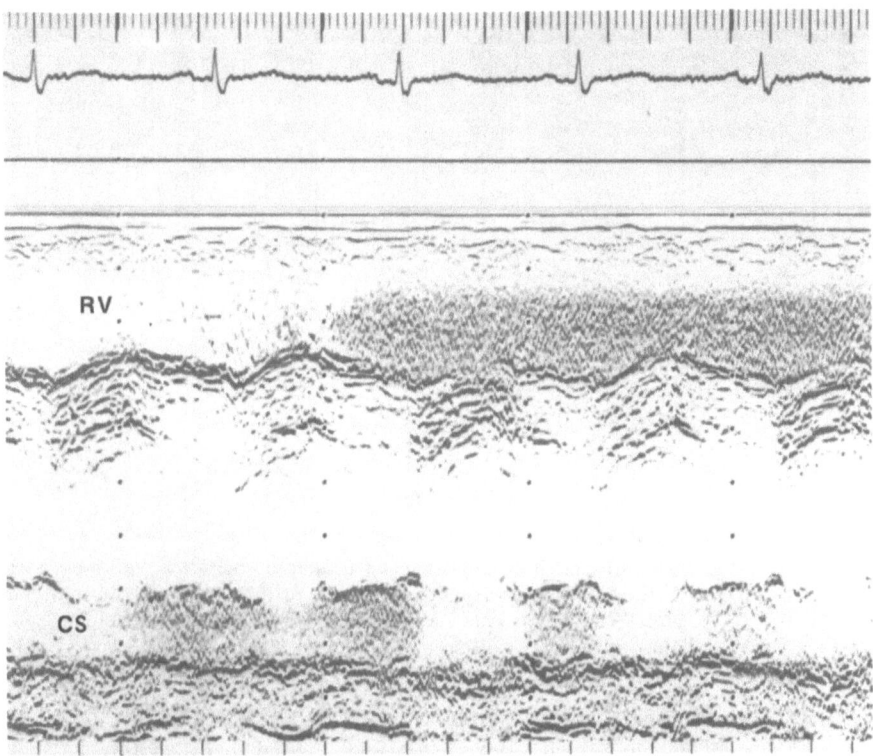

Fig. 4-19 Contrast study showing opacification of the coronary sinus
followed by that of the right ventricle

4.1.4. Ebstein's Anomaly

A) *Anatomy:*

The basic abnormality is a malposition of the tricuspid leaflets with one or more, especially the septal, located nearer the apex within the right ventricular chamber. This results in "atrialisation" of part of the right ventricle and abnormalities of the tricuspid leaflets, commissures and chordae. The valve is functionally stenosed and/or incompetent. ASD with a right-left shunt is usually associated.

Many other cardiac malformations may also be associated, especially type B Wolff-Parkinson-White syndrome[198].

B) *Diagnostic signs:*

M mode: The echo of the anterior tricuspid leaflet is typically very easily recorded, often as soon as the transducer is placed in the usual left parasternal position. The amplitude of motion of this leaflet is very large; it comes into contact with the anterior right ventricular wall echos in diastole and the EF slope is usually reduced (fig. 4-20). The two atrioventricular valves may be recorded simultaneously, and delayed closure of the tricuspid valve diagnosed.

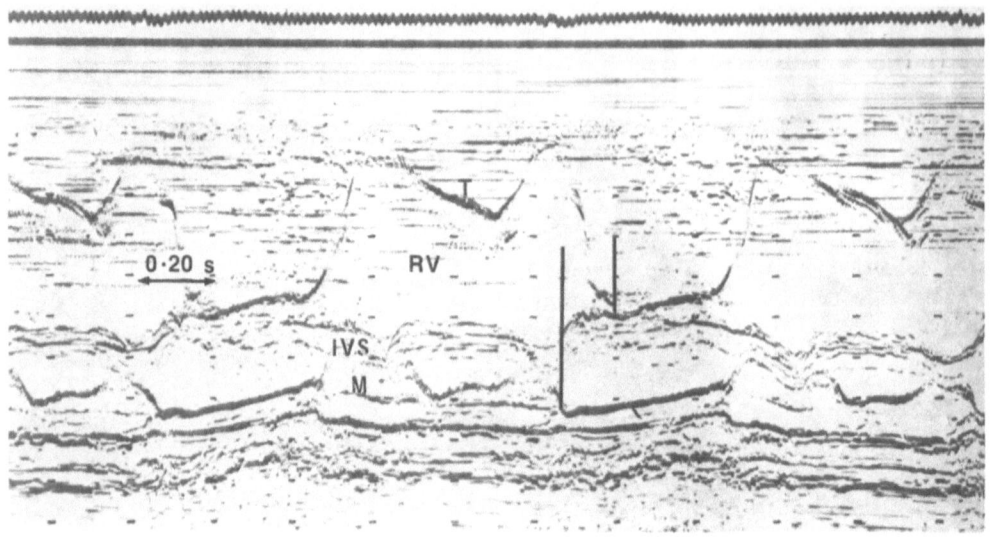

Fig. 4-20 Echocardiogram of simultaneous tricuspid and mitral valve echos in a case of Ebstein's anomaly: the amplitude of the tricuspid valve is abnormally large, the EF slope is reduced and, above all, delayed closure 0·12 sec after mitral valve closure is observed (recorded at 100mm/sec)

Normally, the tricuspid valve closes less than 0.03 seconds after the mitral valve in the absence of right bundle branch block; in Ebstein's anomaly, the closure is delayed 0.04 to 0.12 seconds after mitral closure. If the delay is greater than 0.06 sec., the diagnosis should be strongly suspected[128] [198].

Other non-specific signs may also be recorded: an increased right ventricular internal dimension with variable degrees of paradoxical septal motion (fig. 4-21).

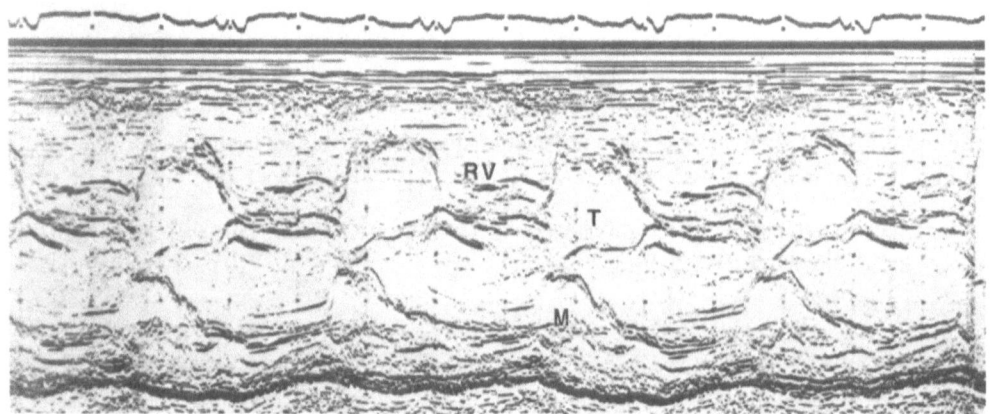

Fig. 4-21 Ebstein's anomaly

2D: The diagnosis is confirmed by the visualisation of the malposition of the origin of the tricuspid valve in the apical 4 chamber view which visualises both atrioventricular valves simultaneously. The insertion of the septal tricuspid leaflet is seen much closer to the apex than that of the mitral leaflet (fig. 4-22) (fig. 4-22 bis)

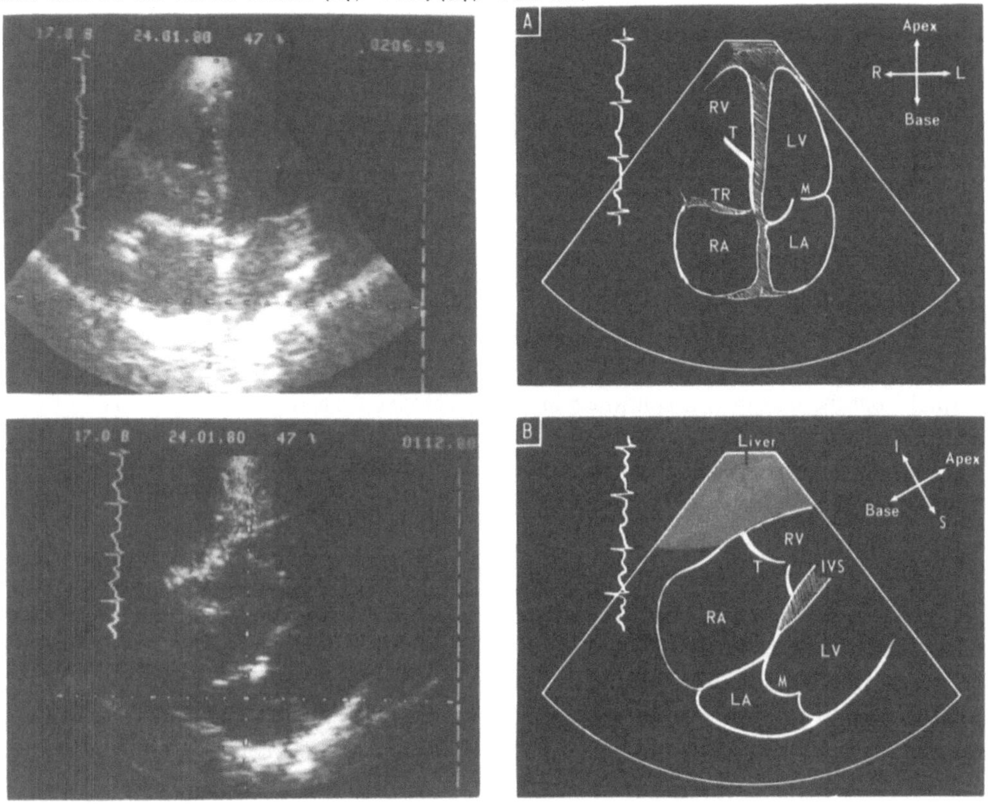

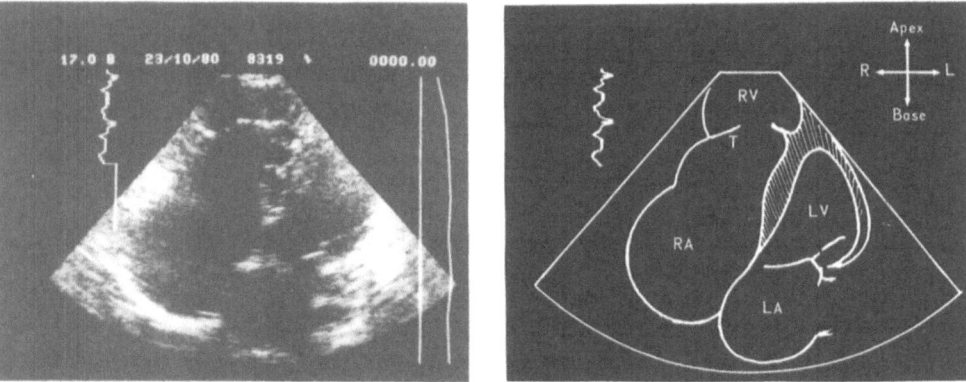

Fig. 4-22 Ebstein's anomaly   A- 2D 4 chamber apical view showing the normal position of the tricuspid ring but the septal tricuspid leaflet has an abnormally low insertion near the apex   B- 2D subcostal view

Fig. 4-22 bis Ebstein's anomaly. Apical 4 chamber view
The tricuspid insertion is displaced downwards and a large zone of the RV is continuous with the right atrium

The tricuspid ring is often in place, realising two right atrial cavities with a rather small functional right ventricular chamber[161]. On the other hand, a dilated anterior chamber with a mobile anterior tricuspid leaflet and a relatively reduced left ventricular internal dimension are recorded from the left parasternal position.

Contrast technique may be used to demonstrate a right-left atrial shunt and the presence of tricuspid incompetence[124]

C) *Diagnostic pitfalls and comments:*

The abnormal lefward displacement of the tricuspid valve should not be confused with the mitral valve. This mistake can be avoided by careful scanning to determine the exact anatomical relationship of these structures.

Depending of the anatomic varieties, the echocardiographic appearances are not always as typical as those described above: the tricuspid valve echos and tricuspid closure may be normal[45] but the diagnosis is confirmed on 2D apical views, vearing out others causes of right diastolic overload.

4.1.5. Uhl's Anomaly (Paper-thin Right Ventricle)

A) *Anatomy:*

This is a rare condition but the incidence appears to be increasing with the recognition of minor forms. The underlying abnormality is a variable degree of agenesis of the right ventricular myocardium. Uhl's first description in 1950 was of a neonate with a major form with right ventricular failure[208]. However, partial forms are often present with cardiac arrhythmias (right ventricular tachycardia). Dilatation of the pulmonary infundibulum is present in all forms of the anomaly.

B) *Diagnostic signs:*

M-mode: the appearances depend on the severity of the condition, but in typical cases, right ventricular diastolic overload[120] with signs suggestive of right ventricular failure (premature pulmonary valve opening, delayed tricuspid closure) are recorded[62] (fig. 4-23).

2D: shows dilatation of the right heart cavities without tricuspid valve malposition and an intact interatrial septum. Contrast techniques exclude intracardiac shunts but may show tricuspid incompetence.

C) *Diagnostic pitfalls and comments:*

No specific echocardiographic sign of this condition has yet been described. Diagnosis is made by eliminating other causes of right ventricular diastolic overload.

In our experience, the pulmonary infundibulum was dilated in all cases, and 2D echo in 3 cases, showed very unusual appearances of the diaphragmatic wall of the right ventricle (in subcostal view): dense (brilliant), thin and immobile. Further study is necessary to confirm this sign.

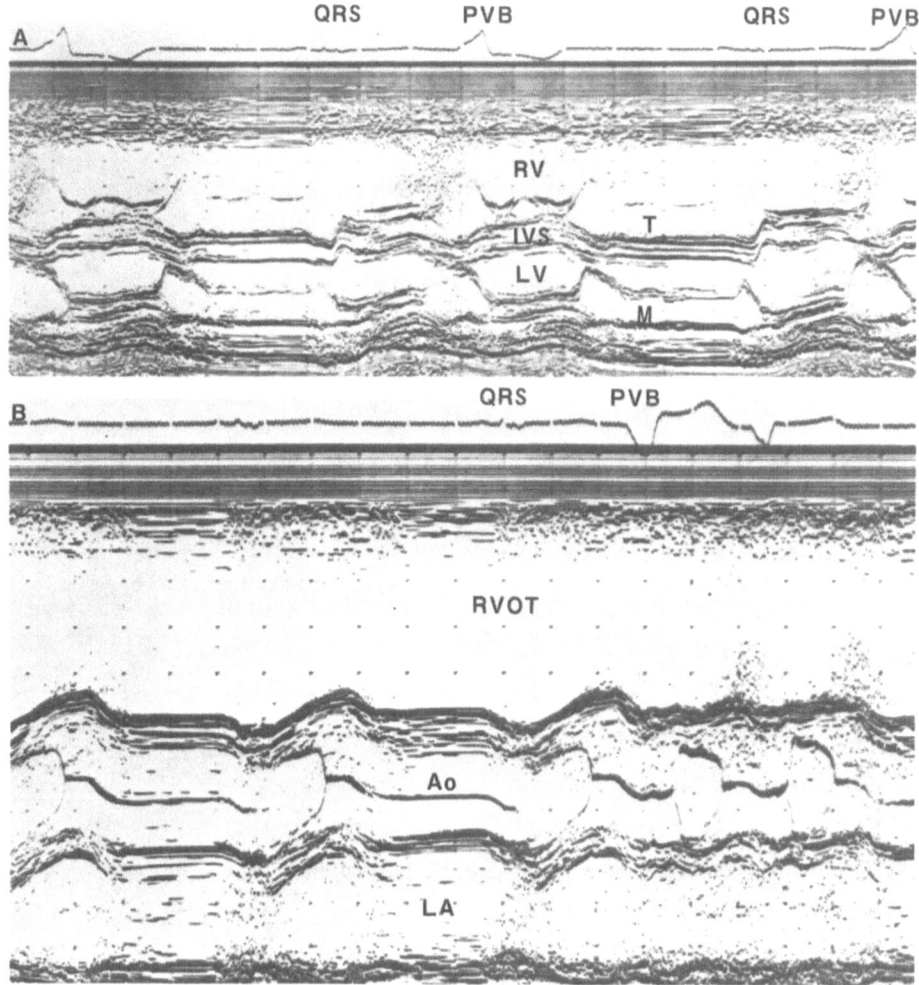

Fig. 4 -23 Uhl's anomaly showing signs of right ventricular diastolic overload (A) and dilatation of the pulmonary infundibulum (B)

4.1.6. Other Causes

Tricuspid incompetence (TI) and pulmonary incompetence (PI) are rarely isolated anomalies and are usually associated with other malformations:

— TI: Direct signs include systolic prolapse and ruptured chordae. Contrast studies show systolic reflux into the inferior vena cava, the diameter of which is increased. Ther is little respiratory variation, and a "to-and-fro" appearance across the tricuspid orifice is observed.

— PI: occurs in severe pulmonary hypertension and after surgery on the pulmonary infundibulum (Fallot's tetralogy, pulmonary stenosis). M-mode echo may show diastolic fluttering of the tricuspid valve[77] (fig. 4-24).

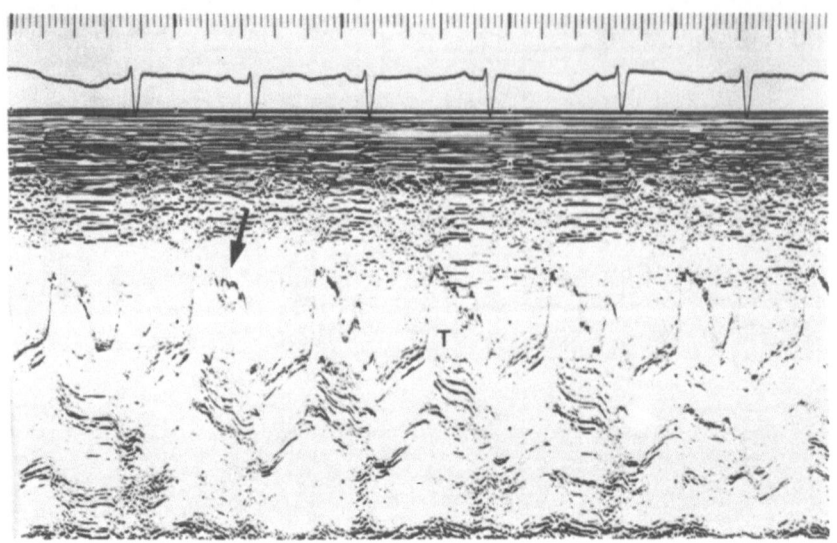

Fig. 4-24 Tricuspid valve echogram in a patient after correction of Fallot's tetralogy showing fine fluttering of the anterior leaflet as a result of pulmonary incompetence

4.2. OBSTRUCTIVE ABNORMALITIES OF THE RIGHT HEART

4.2.1. Valvular pulmonary stenosis

A) *Anatomy:*

This is a common abnormality. There is a variable degree of cusp fusion leading to a dome-like systolic appearance with a small circular hole at the centre. The valve may be bicuspid with a normal or atretic valve ring.

It is frequently associated with ASD, VSD or a more complex malformation (see further on).

B) *Diagnostic signs:*

M-mode : There are no specific signs, but an increased amplitude of the inspiratory pulmonary A wave is suggestive of the diagnosis. Weyman et al[223]. found transvalvular pressure gradients of between 50 and 140 mm Hg in patients with pulmonary A waves of between 8 and 13 mm amplitude (fig. 4-25). In addition, in patients with gradients greater than 65 mm Hg the pulmonary echo did not return to its original position before systolic opening (fig. 4-26). Right ventricular hypertrophy is associated.

2D : It is sometimes possible to record the dome-appearance of the valve, but a thickened valve may occasionally be observed[230].

C) *Diagnostic pitfalls and comments:*

The depth of the A wave must be measured in inspiration. Considerable physiological variations occur during the respiratory cycle. A constant presystolic opening is good evidence for pulmonary stenosis, but can be present in others conditions[62] [128] [229].

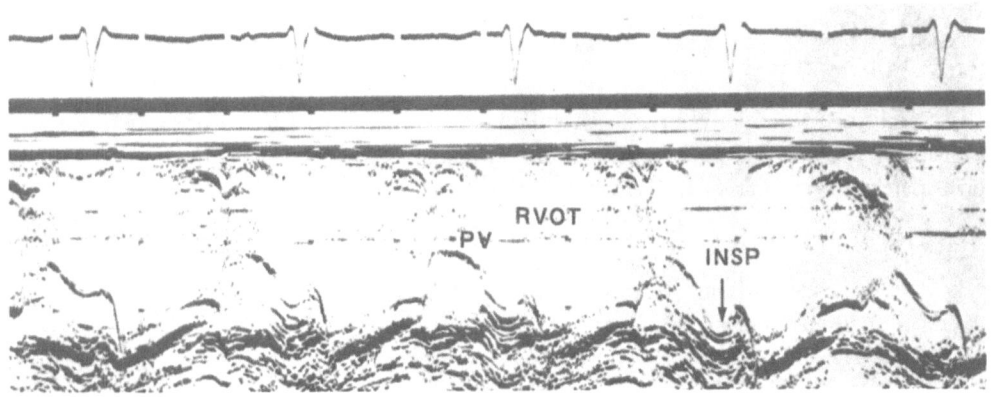

Fig. 4-25 Pulmonary valve in pulmonary stenosis showing variation in the depth of the "a" wave during the respiratory cycle. The maximum depth (arrowed) was measured during inspiration

In mild pulmonary stenosis with pressure gradients less than 50 mm Hg, the A wave is usually normal[229].

Another point to be born in mind is that the depht of the A wave may vary according to the incidence of the ultrasound beam. Finally, aortic root motion strongly influences the pulmonary valve echos and recent publications suggest that the study of the pulmonary valve echo is of little value in this condition[158].

Post operative echo studies show persistence of deep A waves, and, in some cases, signs of pulmonary incompetence.

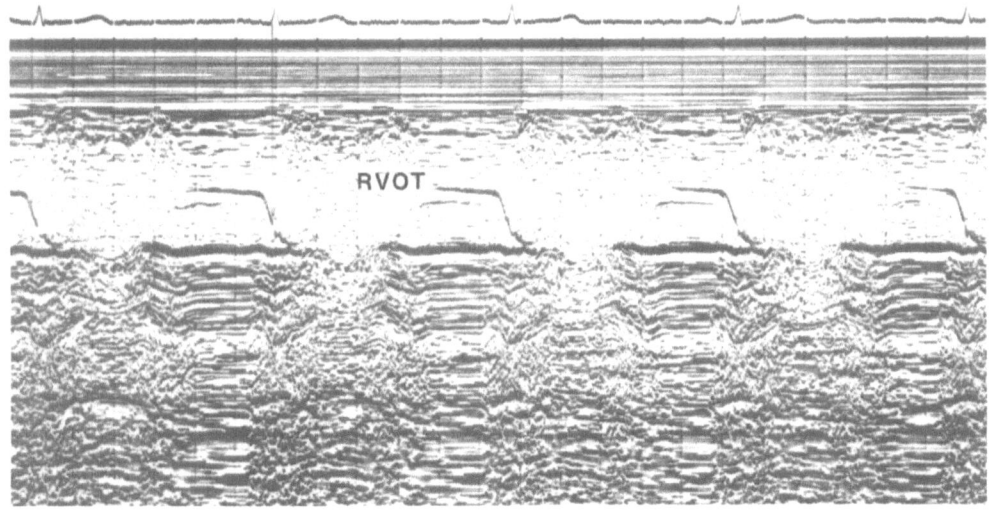

Fig. 4-26 Pulmonary valve in pulmonary stenosis showing constant premature opening

4.2.2. Infundibular pulmonary stenosis

A) *Anatomy:*

Stenosis of the right ventricular outflow tract is rarely an isolated malformation and may be secondary to valvular pulmonary stenosis, or pulmonary hypertension. However, it usually forms part of more complex malformations such as Fallot's tetralogy.

B) *Diagnostic signs:*

M-mode : the striking finding is coarse systolic fluttering of the pulmonary valve; in severe infundibular stenosis the A wave may be absent (in the absence of associated valvular stenosis)[225] (fig. 4-27).

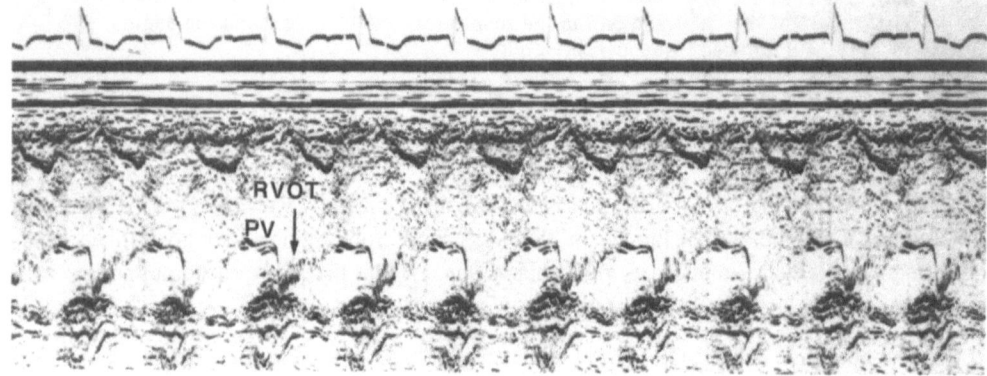

Fig. 4-27 Pulmonary valve echogram from a patient with infundibular pulmonary stenosis

2D: there is a good correlation between angiography and 2D studies of the pulmonary infundibulum in Fallot's tetralogy[16]. The same techniques may be used in isolated infundibular stenosis.

C) *Diagnostic pitfalls and comments:*

Systolic fluttering of the pulmonary valve may be recorded in low output syndromes but without signs of associated right ventricular hypertrophy, and also in pulmonary hypertension, but in this case an increase in the right ventricular preejection period and in the ratio of the preejection period to right ventricular ejection time, is observed[92].

It is a very difficult diagnosis to make on echocardiography, and it does not yet seem possible to quantitate its severity.

A) **Pulmonary atresia with intact ventricular septum**

A) *Anatomy:*

The pulmonary valve is replaced by a closed fibrous diaphragm and as a result the right ventricular cavity and the tricuspid valve are hypoplasic. The size of the ventricle depends on the presence of tricuspid incompetence. For survival, there must be an anatomical or functional ASD (right-left shunt).

B) *Diagnostic signs :*

M-mode : The finding of a small hypoplastic anterior chamber, a small tricuspid valve and the absence of pulmonary valve echos, strongly suggest the diagnosis in a cyanosed neonate. The left heart chambers are rather dilated but the valves and anatomical continuities are normal[50] [135].

2D : The same anatomical signs are confirmed. The use of simultaneous M-mode facilitates recording of hypoplastic tricuspid valve and helps to confirm the absence of a pulmonary valve .

Contrast studies demonstrate the ASD, the patency of the tricuspid orifice and exclude VSD. A better assessment of the geometry of the right ventricle is obtained by using different transducer positions.

C) *Diagnostic pitfalls and comments :*

Hypoplasia of the anterior chamber and of the tricuspid valve makes it difficult to distinguish the interventricular septum from the anterior wall of the right ventricle: its presence excludes the diagnosis of single ventricle with a single atrioventricular valve or left ventricular hypoplasia. It is easier to visualise with 2D echo. Tricuspid atresia with intact interventricular septum gives practically the same echo and clinical appearances, but they may be distinguished by the presence of tricuspid valve echos.

B) Tricuspid Atresia

A) *Anatomy :*

Imperforation or agenesis of the tricuspid valve is associated with a right-left shunt at atrial level. The size of the right ventricle depends on the presence and size of an associated VSD; in cases of intact septum the right ventricle is vestigial, whilst in cases of VSD the pulmonary infundibulum is more developed, especially when transposition of the great vessels is associated (common).

B) *Diagnostic signs :*

Tricuspid atresia with intact interventricular septum has been discussed above. The signs of tricuspid atresia with VSD are described below.

M-mode : Besides careful scanning to confirm the absence of a tricuspid valve, the size of the right ventricular cavity is particularly important: hypoplasia is associated with a poor prognosis[74]. The left heart chambers are dilated[108] [186]. It is also important to search for a pulmonary valve, to assess pulmonary hypertension and to analyse the relationships of the great vessels to exclude transposition.

2D : and contrast echo are indispensable in the evaluation of the right ventricle and its outflow tract (on which the surgical possibilities depend), of the size of the VSD, and they also help detect transposition[188] (fig. 4-28).

The specific sign is absence of tricuspid valve echos, a difficult negative sign to confirm by M-mode or 2D echo; the flow of contrast from RA → LA → LV (via mitral valve) → RV outflow tract is diagnostic[180].

Fig. 4-28
Tricuspid
atresia

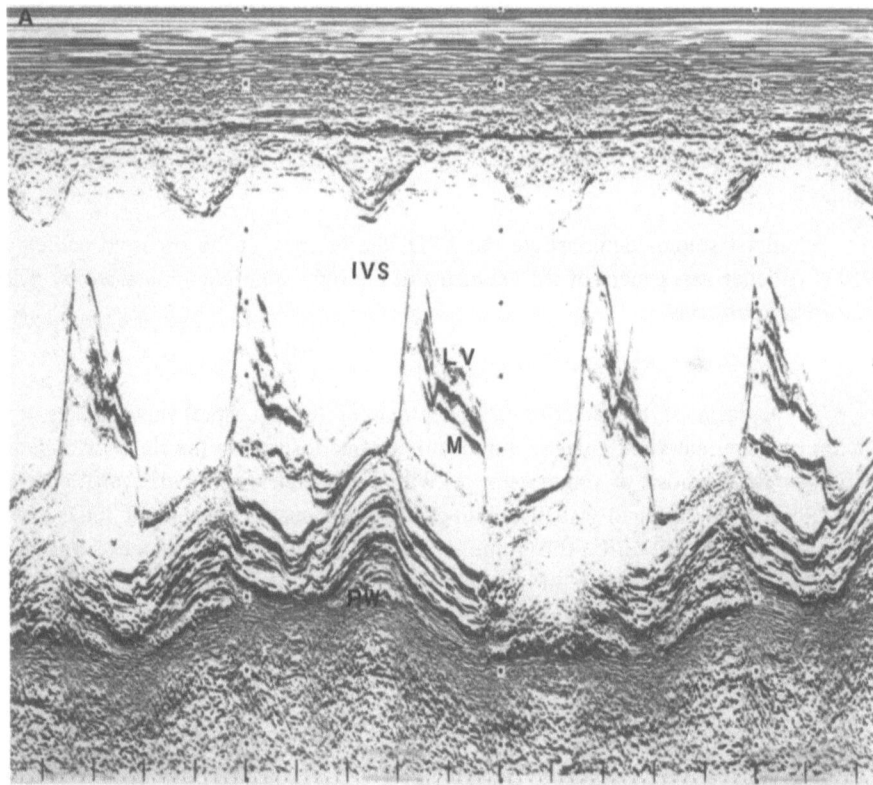

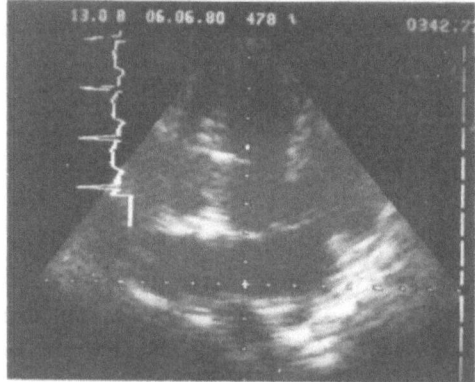
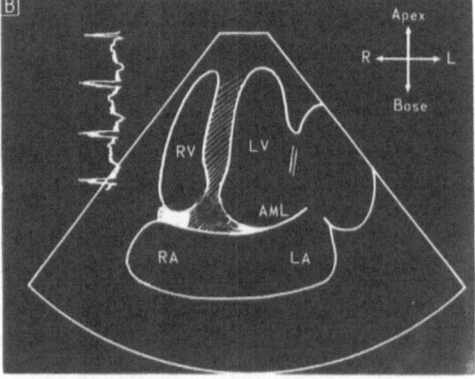

A- Mmode: LV dilatation. The RV cavity cannot be defined. The mitral valve echos are thickened and have a large amplitude of excursion

B- 2D: apical 4 chamber view systolic frame. LV dilatation is confirmed. The RV is hypoplastic and the echos of the tricuspid ring are very dense; the tricuspid leaflets are not visualised

CHAPTER 5

LEFT HEART MALFORMATIONS

5.1. LEFT VENTRICULAR VOLUME OVERLOAD

These malformations all give rise to left ventricular dilatation with normal left ventricular function, so distinguishing them from the cardiomyopathies, and a normal h/r ratio. The wall movement is often hyperdynamic (fig. 5-1) and the left atrium may be dilated (except in cases of pure aortic incompetence). In M mode, the right ventricle can appear to be small as it is displaced behind the septum by the left ventricular dilatation.

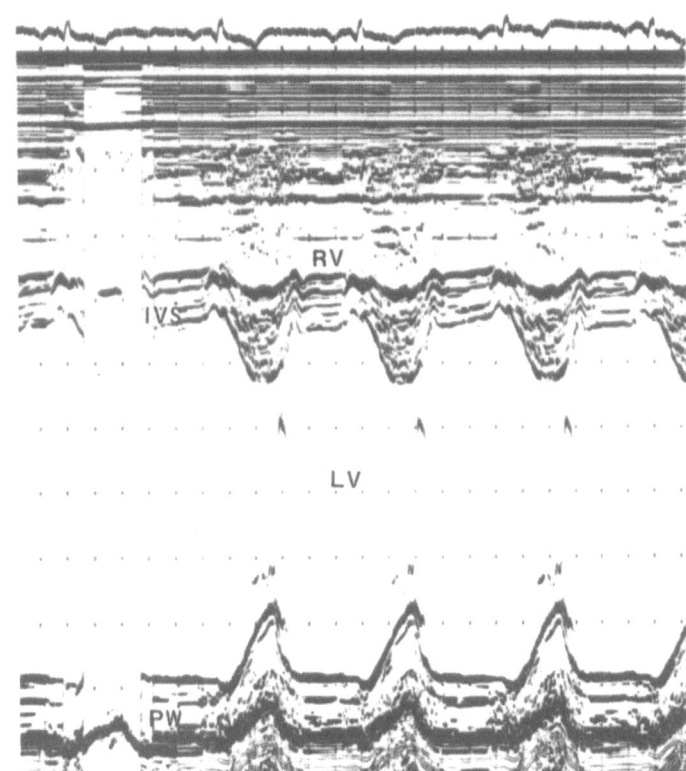

Fig. 5-1
M mode echocardiogram in a patient with VSD showing left ventricular volume overload

5.1.1. Ventricular septal defect (VSD)

This condition often forms part of a more complex malformation. Only isolated VSD will be described in this chapter.

A) *Anatomy :*

The defect may be situated in several sites (membranous septum, within parietal band, near the insertion of the septal leaflet of the tricuspid valve and in the muscular part of the septum). It results in a left to right shunt between the ventricles, or more rarely, between the

101

left ventricle and right atrium. The defect is usually small; large shunts may cause pulmonary hypertension.

B) *Diagnostic signs:*

— *M mode:* It is exceptionally rare to visualise the VSD directly and in small shunts the appearances may be completely normal. However, in larger shunts, signs of left ventricular volume overload compatible with but not specific for VSD are recorded. Septal motion is normal in the absence of complications.

An increased left atrial diameter is considered to be a sign of increased pulmonary blood flow; when the LA/AO ratio is compared to the shunt volume (QP/QS ratio) a linear correlation is obtained (r = 0,96). This allows an assessment of the haemodynamic conditions, even if pulmonary arterial resistance is increased[123]. A normal LA/AO ratio excludes a significant shunt[171].

— *2D:* direct visualisation of the VSD is facilitated by varying the position of the transducer[18] (fig. 5-2). In our experience, contrast studies have not been diagnostic but they do allow exclusion of a right to left shunt.

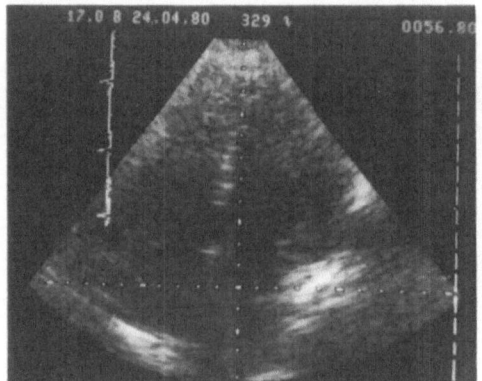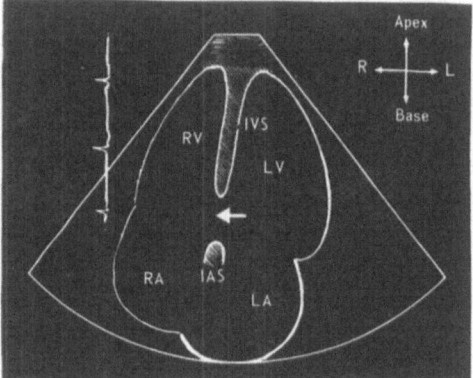

Fig. 5-2 2D four-chamber view in a patient with VSD (arrowed)

C) *Diagnostic pitfalls and comments:*

Its is not possible to distinguish between patent ductus and VSD with M mode echo, but the shunt volume may be estimated. However, systolic fluttering of the tricuspid valve is suggestive of a LV-RA communication[146].

Repeated echocardiography is useful in the follow-up of these patients:

— The appearance of an aneurysm of the membranous septum is suggestive of progressive closure of a VSD[176] (fig. 5-3).

— Repeated study of pulmonary systolic time intervals may detect increasing pulmonary arterial resistance[92].

— The patch may be visualised on post operative studies as an echo brighter than septum

(2D) and normalisation of the cavity sizes may be followed.

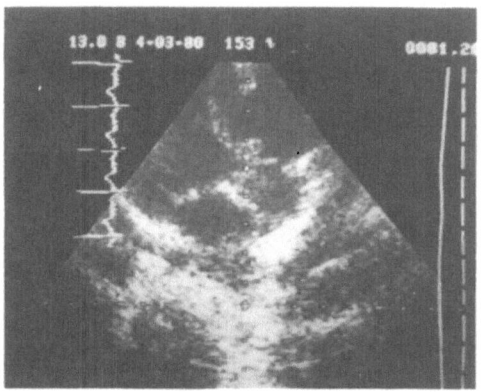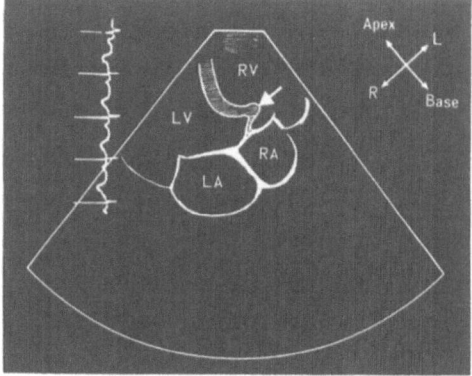

Fig. 5-3 2D apical view showing an anevrysm of the interventricular septum (arrowed): the right heart chambers are displayed on the right

5.1.2. Patent ductus arteriosus (PDA)

A) *Anatomy:*

This abnormality results from persistance of the sixth aortic arch which during foetal life joins the left pulmonary artery to the descending thoracic aorta. The shunt is normally left to right unless pulmonary vascular resistance is raised. The malformation may be associated with any other form of congenital heart disease. There is a higher incidence in premature babies, as its closure is delayed by hypoxia and acidosis, and it may give rise to cardiac failure.

B) *Diagnostic signs:*

— *M mode:* the only changes are the indirect signs of left ventricular overload. As in VSD, the LA/AO ratio gives an estimation of shunt volume and the study of right ventricular systolic time intervals an assessment of pulmonary vascular resistance[187].

— *2D:* Sahn has recently shown that it is possible in some cases to visualise the PDA directly by following the pulmonary artery echos[173] (fig. 5-3 bis).

C) *Diagnostic pitfalls and comments:*

In practice, it is difficult to differentiate between VSD and PDA, without the clinical context. Sahn's publication is exceptional and the absence of the appearances he described, in no way excludes the diagnosis. Aorto-pulmonary window gives the same echocardiographic and clinical signs. The closure of PDA is accompanied by a reduction in left atrial size and this may also be observed after surgical ligature.

5.1.3. Other causes

These include aortic and mitral incompetence which will be discussed in the chapter on valvular heart disease.

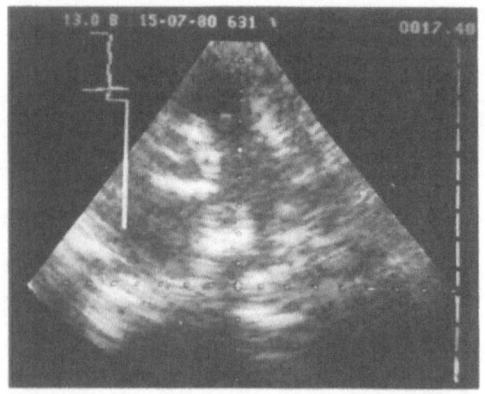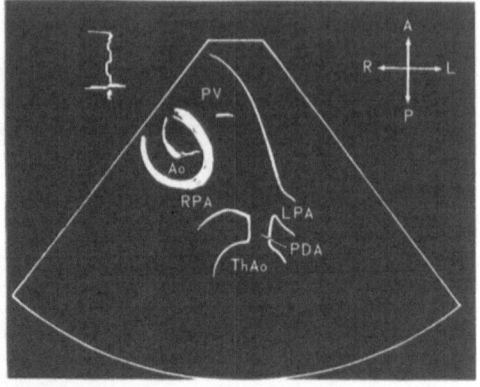

Fig. 5-3 bis Patent ductus arteriosus (PDA) short axis view of the base of the heart. The ductus is visualised between the left pulmonary artery (LPA) and the thoracic aorta (ThAo)

5.2. OBSTACLES TO LEFT VENTRICULAR EJECTION

The echocardiographic signs common to these malformations result from left ventricular pressure overload and lead to symmetric parietal hypertrophy with normal or reduced left ventricular internal dimensions[80] (fig. 5-7). The hypertrophy is a reflection of left ventricular systolic stress, and, based on this hypothesis, several workers[5] [8] [67] have shown that it may be possible to deduce the intraventricular systolic pressure, providing heart failure and associated regurgitant lesions are excluded.

$$LVSP = \frac{SW_T}{LVID_S} \times 225$$

LVSP = left ventricular systolic pressure in mm Hg
SW_T = systolic thickness of the posterior wall
$LVID_S$ = left ventricular systolic internal diameter

This formula, which is deduced of the law of Laplace, gives excellent echo-haemodynamic correlations in children. By taking the systemic blood pressure at arm it therefore becomes possible to estimate the ventriculo-aortic pressure gradient[5] [67].

The systolic stress may also be assessed by measuring the diastolic wall thickness and by the h/r ratio but the published correlations are less satisfactory[8]. Wall hypertrophy (LV mass) remains unchanged in the immediate postoperative period. However, when it persists after one year, a significant residual gradient should be suspected[67]. Serial echocardiograms are a useful mean of pre and post operative assessment, so decreasing the need for cardiac catheterisation.

The obstacles are located at three levels:

— The left ventricular outflow tract: hypertrophic obstructive cardiomyopathy (which will be described in the chapter on cardiomyopathy) and subvalvular stenosis.

— Valvular aortic stenosis.

— Supravalvular aortic stenosis and coarctation.

Contrast studies are only useful for the detection of certain types of associated malformations.

5.2.1. Subvalvular stenosis

A) Anatomy:

Three types of subvalvular stenosis may be identified[142]:

— thin subvalvular membrane stenosis;

— fibromuscular tunnelar stenosis of the outflow tract;

— subvalvular fibrous ring stenosis.

The anterior mitral leaflet may be involved in any of these types of subvalvular obstruction. Jet lesions of the aortic cusps are common and lead to moderate regurgitation.

Coarctation of the aorta and VSD are often associated and all types of congenital anomaly of the mitral valve may also occur.

B) Diagnostic signs:

— M mode: All types of subvalvular stenosis give rise to changes of the aortic valve echos: early systolic closure of one or two cusps followed by partial reopening. This is associated with marked coarse systolic fluttering[35][110][116] (fig. 5-4).

Fig. 5-4
Aortic valve echogram in discrete subaortic stenosis showing early systolic closure

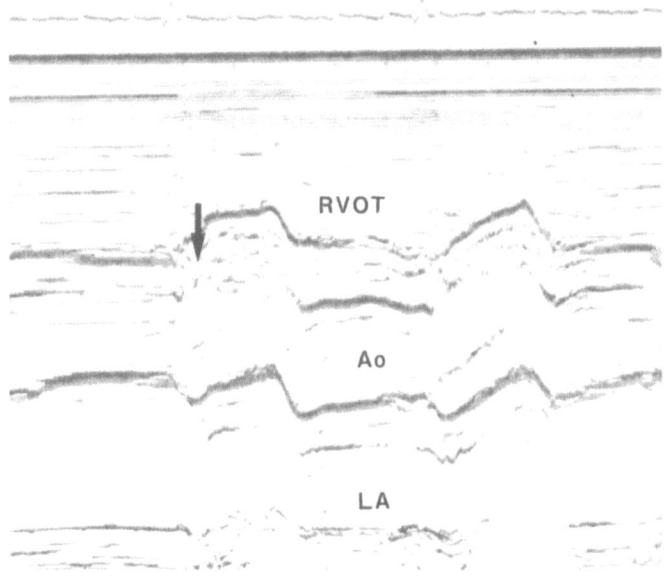

105

• In membranous subvalvular stenosis, an abnormal, thin echo in the left ventricular outflow tract, which may be continuous with the echo of the anterior mitral leaflet, giving rise to appearances similar to those of systolic anterior motion of the mitral valve, may be recorded[116].

• In fibromuscular tunnel stenosis, the dimension of the left ventricular outflow tract is seen to be much smaller than that of the aorta with septal thickening due to fibromuscular infiltration[110].

• In fibrous ring stenosis any combination of the signs described above may be observed (fig. 5-5).

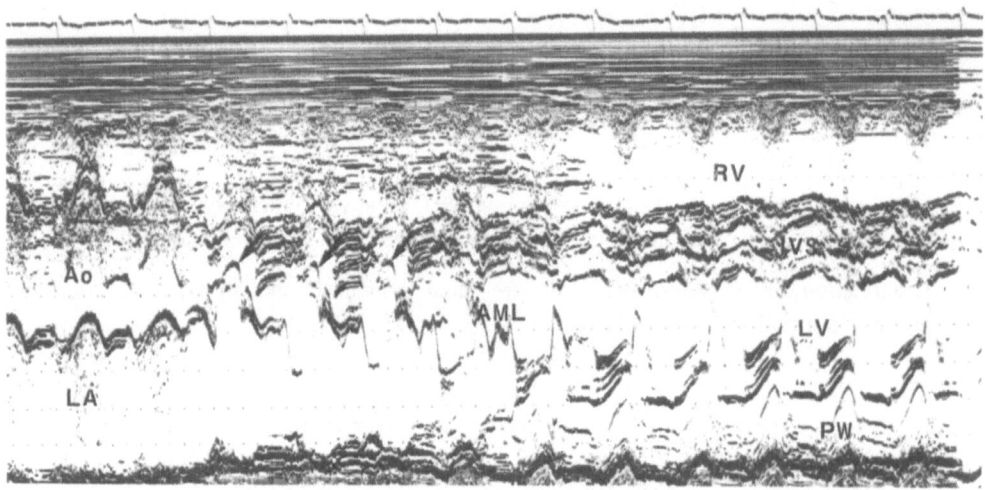

Fig. 5-5   M mode scan of a patient with membranous subaortic stenosis. The membrane is shown (↗) in the left ventricular outflow tract. Diastolic fluttering of the anterior mitral leaflet and infiltration of the subaortic portion of the interventricular septum may also be observed

• Diastolic fluttering of the mitral valve is a sign of associated aortic incompetence.

— 2D: The long axis view (fig. 5-6) gives the anatomical diagnosis plus information on the level of stenosis and the presence of associated mitral valve lesions[227]. The cross-sectional area of the left ventricular outflow tract may be measured by planimetry on transverse views.

C) *Diagnostic pitfalls and comments:*

Early systolic closure of the aortic valve is observed in other pathologies. In hypertrophic obstructive cardiomyopathy, it tends to occur a little later in systole; asymmetric septal hypertrophy and systolic anterior motion of the mitral valve are associated[87].

This sign is frequently encountered to a lesser degree, when a "third space" exists (mitral incompetence, VSD, ventricular aneurysm)[109].

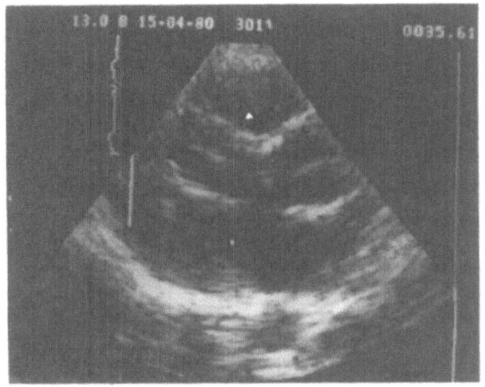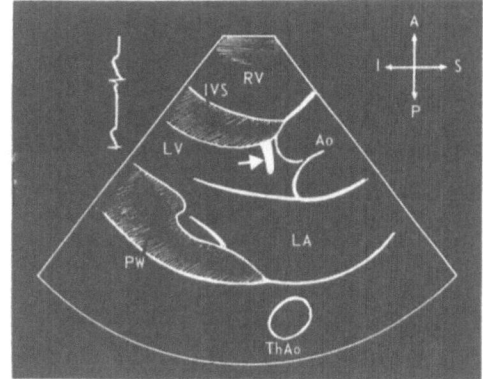

Fig. 5-6 2D long axis view. Diastolic frame in a patient with membranous subaortic stenosis. The insertion of the membrane into the upper interventricular septum is shown (⤴)

Abnormal echos in the left ventricular outflow tract may suggest aortic cusp prolapse with or without regurgitation but, in this case, the echos are only recorded in diastole.

Septal infiltration may suggest asymmetric septal hypertrophy but this condition is usually more diffuse and only rarely affects the subaortic septum alone. It may be difficult to distinguish these two conditions on M mode (in the presence of systolic anterior motion of the mitral valve), especially as the two may be associated[109], but 2D echo is the key to the diagnosis[227].

5.2.2. Congenital valvular aortic stenosis

A) *Anatomy:*

The aortic orifice is eccentric and reduced by fusion of the commissures. The deformed valve has a domed systolic appearance with one, two (bicuspid valve) or three cusps. The aortic cusps are generally thickened; usually, the valve is bicuspid, but bicuspid valve is not always stenotic. The cusps tend to calcify with time and aortic incompetence and infective endocarditis may complicate the outcome.

Other obstacles to ejection may be associated (coarctation).

B) *Diagnostic signs:*

— *M mode:* The aortic cusps are thin or slightly thickened and usually separate normally in systole. In diastole, multiple parallel echos are often recorded (fig. 5-7). In bicuspid aortic valve, the diastolic echo is eccentrically located: an eccentricity index (half the internal diameter of the aorta divided by the minimum distance from the diastolic echo and the nearest aortic wall) greater than 1,5 is considered diagnostic[143] [163] (fig. 5-8). The aortic diameter is normal or slightly reduced (small aortic ring).

— *2D:* A direct image of the aortic valve in diastole may be obtained with a transverse view (fig. 5-9). The long axis view shows the domed systolic appearance and allows measurement of maximal systolic separation[226] (fig. 5-10)

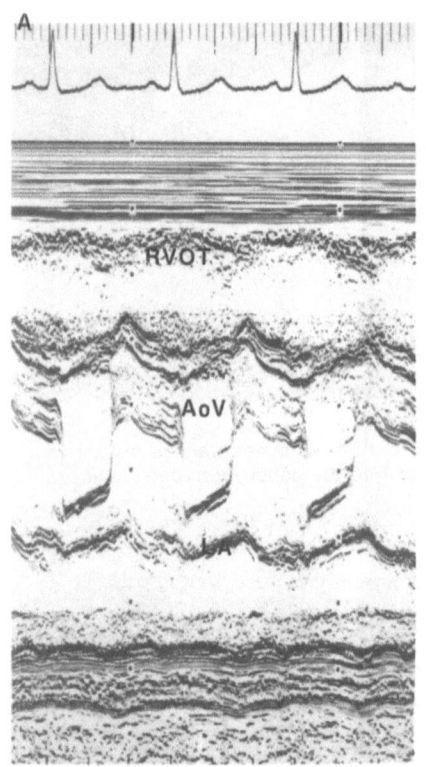

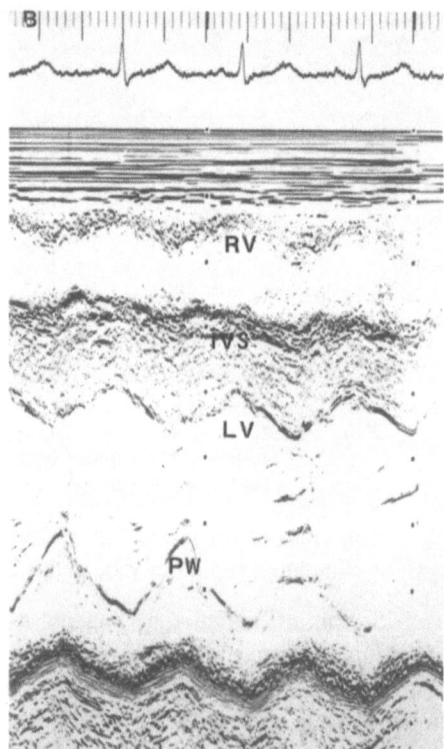

Fig. 5-7
Congenital aortic stenosis
A- The aortic cusps appear
to separate normally in
systole but multiple
echos are recorded in
diastole
B- Symmetric left
ventricular hypertrophy

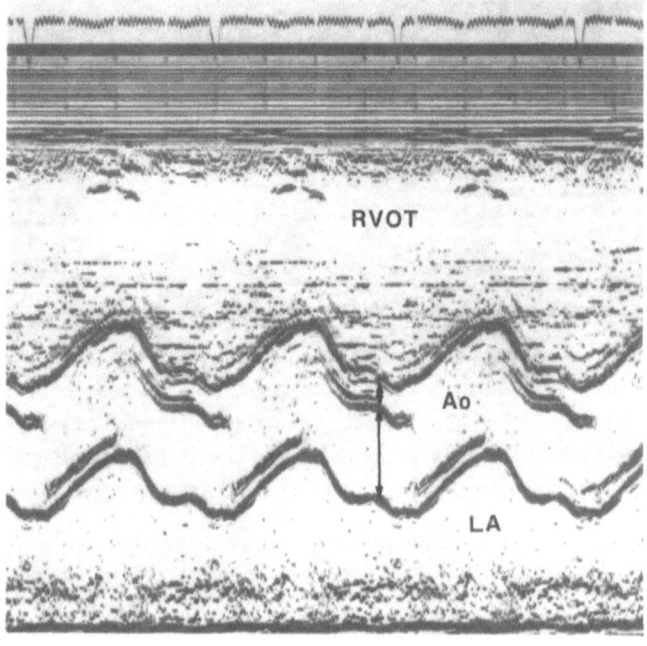

Fig. 5-8
Echocardiogramm in a
case of bicuspid aortic
valve showing the
eccentric diastolic
echos

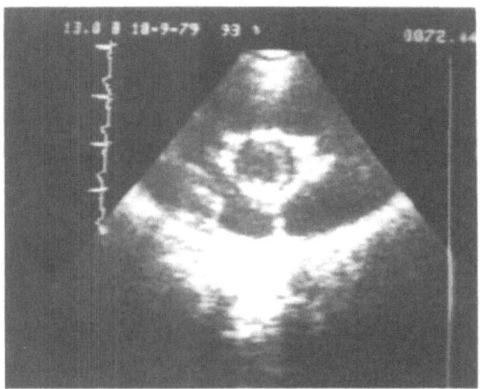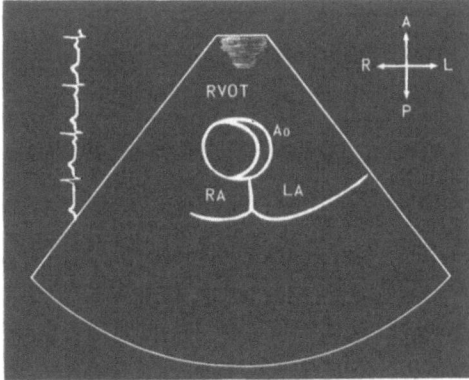

Fig. 5-9 2D short axis view of the base of the heart showing
a bicuspid aortic valve

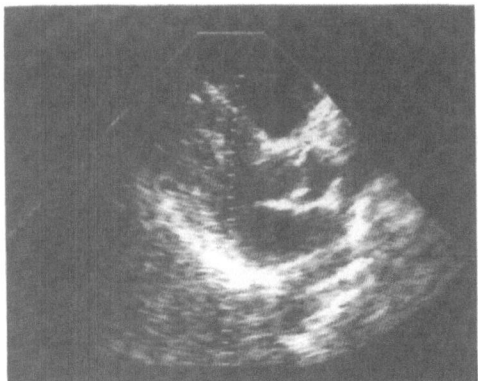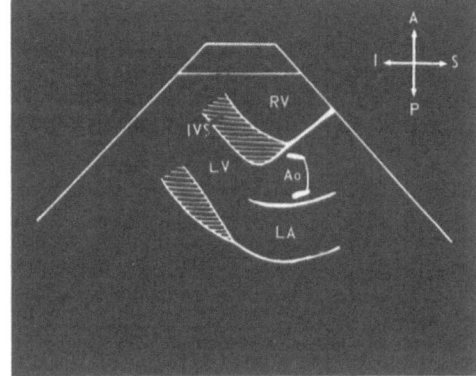

*Fig.5-10 2D long axis view of congenital aortic stenosis showing
the domed appearence of the aortic valve in systole

C) *Diagnostic pitfalls and comments*

Normal M mode appearances of the aortic valve do not exclude congenital aortic stenosis: analysis of left ventricular wall thickness may suggest the possibility of obstruction to ejection.

When an eccentric diastolic echo is found in all incidences of examination, a bicuspid valve is very probable. Otherwise, the diagnosis can only be made by 2D echo.

The diastolic aortic echo may also be eccentric in cases of aneurysm of the sinus of Valsalva[168] (see chapter on Aortic pathology Tome II).

5.2.3. **Supraaortic stenosis**

A) *Anatomy*

This diffuse narrowing of the ascending aorta may form part of a congenital syndrome including hypercalcaemia and mental retardation. It is rare, unlike coarctation which is located at the site of the ductus arteriosus.

In addition to the signs of left ventricular pressure overload, narrowing of the aorta in the supravalvular region, best visualised with 2D echo, is suggestive[211] [231].

In the coarctation the supra sternal view sometimes allows direct visualisation of the lesion[172] [232].

5.3. OBSTRUCTIONS TO FILLING OF THE LEFT HEART

These malformations are very rare and may be located at different sites: the left atrium (cor triatriatum), the left ventricular inflow tract (supra mitral ring), the mitral valve or the papillary muscles. They vary in degrees of severity and may present in adult life. The signs common to all these pathologies are dilatation of the left atrium, with possible pulmonary hypertension and dilatation of the right heart cavities.

5.3.1. Cor triatriatum

A) *Anatomy:*

An anomalous fibro muscular diaphragm separates the left atrium into two cavities, one posteriorly which receives the pulmonary veins and the other anteriorly which contains the left auricle and the mitral ring. This usually is an isolated malformation.

B) *Diagnostic signs*

— *M mode:* The diagnosis is suggested by the presence of an abnormal intra atrial echo, usually situated close to the posterior aortic wall. It has a similar motion and the echos may in fact be in continuity (fig. 5-11). The mitral valve motion is normal[19] [111].

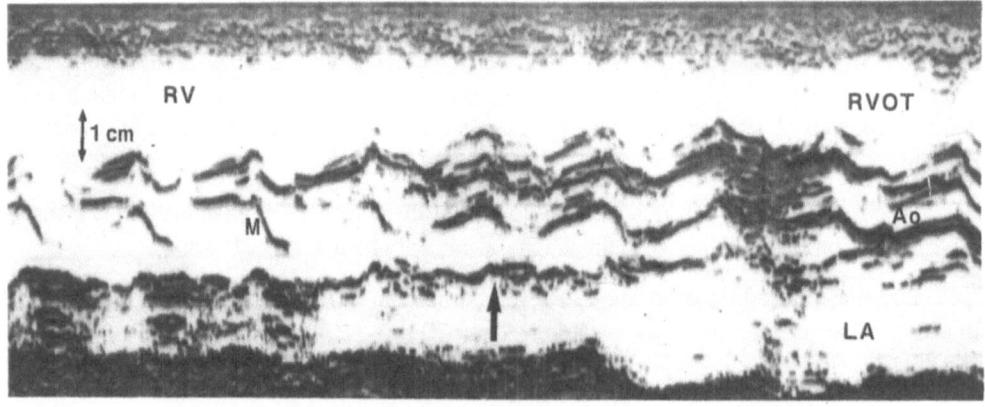

Fig. 5-11 Cor triatriatum in the new born. M mode scan of the aortic root and left atrium showing the mitro-atrial diaphragm

— *2D:* The location of the diaphragm may be determined in the left atrium[167] (fig. 5-12).

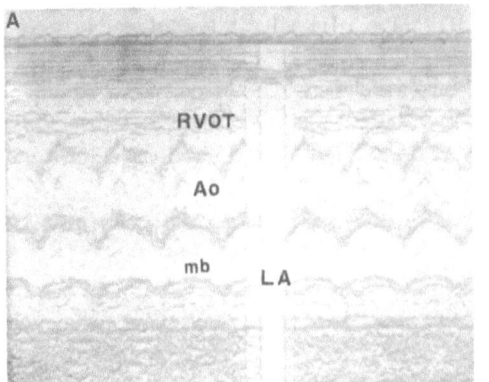
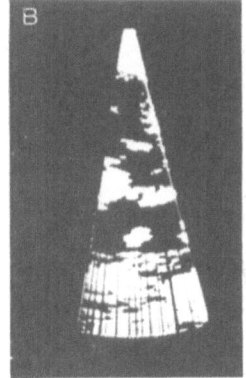
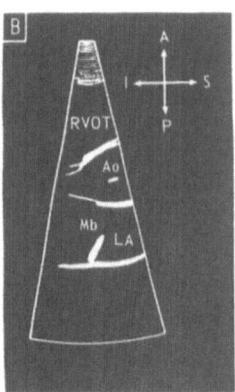

Fig. 5-12   Cor triatriatum in a 23 years old man
A- M mode echocardiogram showing the abnormal echo in the left atrium (Mb) separating it into two chambers
B- A 30° 2D long axis view of the aorta and left atrium showing the position of the membrane

C) *Diagnostic pitfalls and comments*

When the abnormal echo is posteriorly situated on M mode, the diagnosis may be confused with abnormal pulmonary venous return (see APVR). The supravalvular mitral ring may give similar appearances in diastole, but when the mitral leaflets close, the echo merges with the systolic mitral echos. In addition, valvular lesions are always associated[111].

5.3.2. Congenital abnormalities of the mitral apparatus

A) *Anatomy*

These abnormalities may consist of a fibrous supra valvular ring, commisural fusion with varying malformations of the leaflets and chordae, or a single papillary muscle with shortened chordae (parachute deformity). The fibrous ring is always associated with valvular stenosis.

B) *Diagnostic signs:*

— *M mode:* The amplitude of mitral valve opening and its diastolic slope are usually reduced; abnormal anterior diastolic motion of the posterior mitral leaflet is also recorded (fusion of the commissures). The supra valvular ring is sometimes visible in the left atrium[30]. Systolic anterior motion has been described in parachute deformity of the mitral valve[14].

— *2D:* The level of the lesion (supravalvular ring or single papillary muscle) may be determined by short axis views[167] (fig. 5-13).

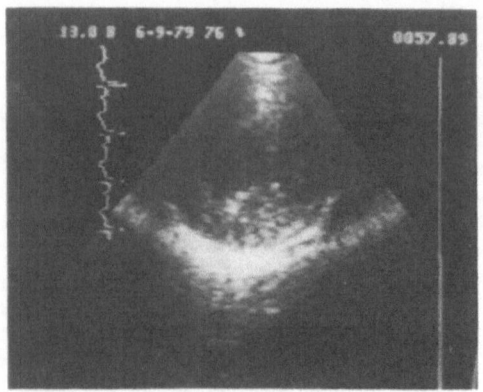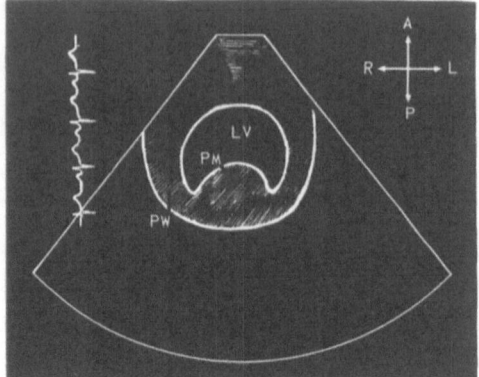

Fig. 5-13 2D short axis view of the left ventricle of a patient with parachute deformity of the mitral valve showing the single large median papillary muscle (PM)

5.4. HYPOPLASIA OF THE LEFT HEART

A) *Anatomy:*

This anatomical syndrome consists of hypoplasia of the left ventricle, atresia or hypoplasia of one or both left heart valves and hypoplasia of the ascending aorta. Systemic blood flow is maintained by a patent ductus arteriosus, closure of which leads to irreversible cardiogenic shock.

B) *Diagnostic signs*[74] [127] [135]:

Careful scanning shows a tiny aorta with an internal dimension of less than 5 mm and a left ventricle with a diastolic internal dimension of less than 1 cm[50bis] [135]. The mitral valve, when present, has a very reduced amplitude of motion[6] [135]. Anteriorly, the right heart cavities are dilated. A large anterior atrioventricular valve and signs of pulmonary hypertension are recorded; the interventricular septum shows paradoxical motion[50bis] [135].

C) *Diagnostic pitfalls and comments:*

The great difficulty in examination and diagnosis lies in the demonstration of an interventricular septum. It lies against the posterior wall and its continuity with the aorta and the presence of a mitral ring or valve confirms the diagnosis of hypoplasia and exclude the different forms of single ventricule. In right ventricular hypoplasia, the same appearances are observed but the septum is very anterior.

Very severe left ventricular hypertrophy, which is absent in hypoplasia, may give rise to small ventricular cavities in severe obstruction to left ventricular ejection, but the conditions may benefit from surgery.

In practice, echocardiography confirms the diagnosis of a hypoplastic left heart, so avoiding the necessity of further investigation[114] [188].

CHAPTER 6
ABNORMALITIES OF THE GREAT ARTERIES

Malposition of the great arteries with respect to the interventricular septum without anatomical continuity is common to all these conditions[217].

6.1. FALLOT'S TETRALOGY. PULMONARY ATRESIA WITH VSD. TRUNCUS ARTERIOSUS

A) *Anatomy:*

These three malformations are characterised by hypoplasia or atresia of the right ventricular outflow tract, a large subaortic VSD, and dilatation and dextro position of the aorta. This consequence is a right to left shunt.

— *Fallot's tetralogy*

This results from an abnormality in the development of the parietal band which is hypertrophied and displaced upwards and to the right, so obstructing the pulmonary outflow tract[216]. This leads to dextro-positioning of the aorta and to a VSD. The pulmonary valve and artery are hypoplastic, the extreme form being *pulmonary atresia with VSD* or pseudo-truncus.

Right ventricular hypertrophy is constant.

— *Truncus arteriosus*

A single great artery arises from the base of the heart and there is complete absence of the pulmonary outflow tract. The number of valve cusps varies between 2 and 6 and sometimes a certain degree of regurgitation is present. The pulmonary arteries are given off the truncus.

B) *Diagnostic signs:*

— *M mode:* The signs common to all three malformations are[2] [22] [29] [63] [117]:

● a large systemic artery overriding the interventricular septum (fig. 6-1);

● normal continuity between the anterior mitral leaflet and the posterior wall of this artery (fig. 6-1);

● right ventricular dilatation and hypertrophy with normal septal motion (fig. 6-2).

The internal dimension of the left atrium gives an idea of the pulmonary blood flow[2]. The presence of diastolic fluttering of the mitral valve is either related to regurgitation (aortic or truncal) or to a diastolic ventricular right to left shunt.

The recording of a pulmonary valve distinguishes Fallot's tetralogy from the other two conditions[29]. It has the same appearances as in subvalvular stenosis (systolic fluttering) and occasionally presystolic opening is observed (valvular stenosis).

The greater the dextro-position of the aorta, the more severe the Fallot[117].

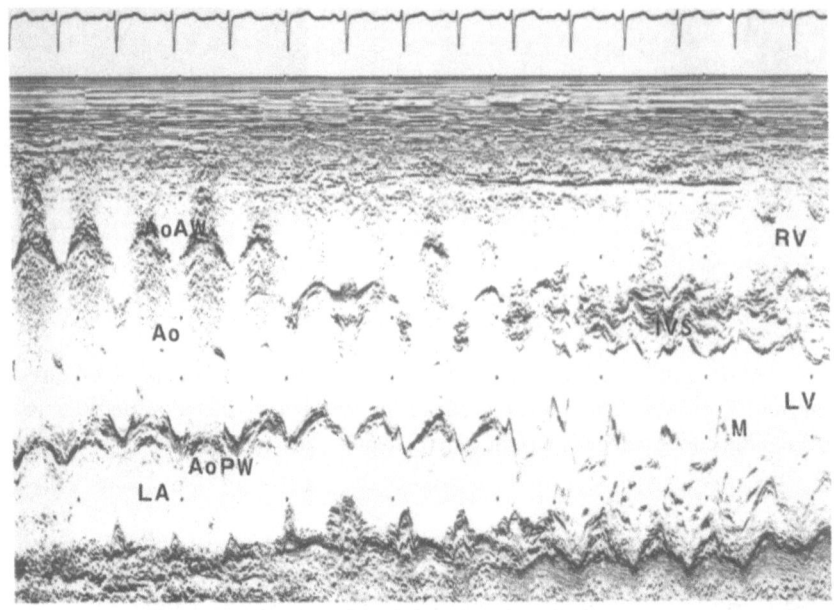

Fig. 6-1

Fallot's tetralogy:
M mode scan showing the dilated aorta
overriding the interventricular septum
giving rise to aorto-septal discontinuity

Fig. 6-2

Fallot's tetralogy:
M mode echocardiogram showing RV
dilatation and severe hypertrophy of
the RV anterior wall and IVS

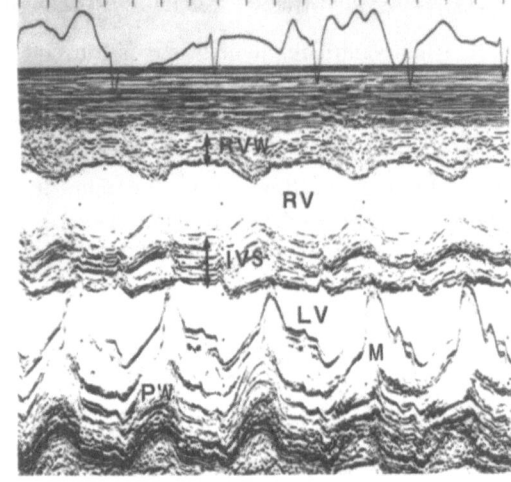

— *2D:* This allows study of the right ventricular outflow tract which is not possible with M mode. The visualisation of two vessels at the base of the heart immediately distinguishes Fallot's tetralogy from Truncus arteriosus[2]. In both cases, the overriding great artery and the VSD are visible on parasternal, apical and subcostal long axis views, so enabling quantification of the degree of dextro position (fig. 6-3, 6-4). The pulmonary valve is recorded on simultaneous M mode from the 2D transverse view of the base of the heart in Fallot's tetralogy. The dimensions of the pulmonary infundibulum may also be measured[16]. Angulating the transducer superiorly brings the bifurcation of the main pulmonary artery and a few centimetres of the right and left pulmonary arteries into the field of vision and localised stenoses may be detected (fig. 6-5).

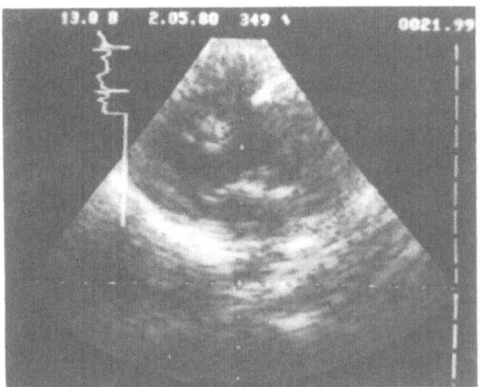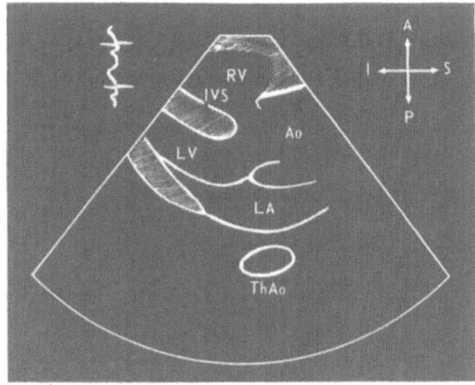

Fig. 6-3 Fallot's tetralogy: long axis view; systolic frame showing overriding of the dilated aorta

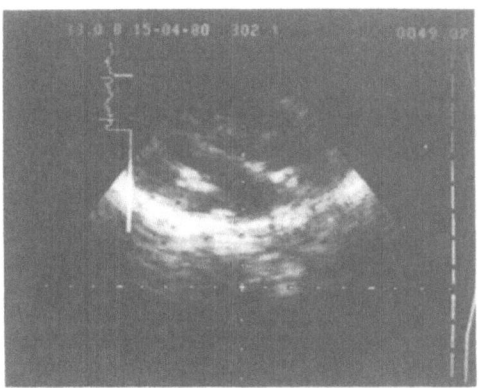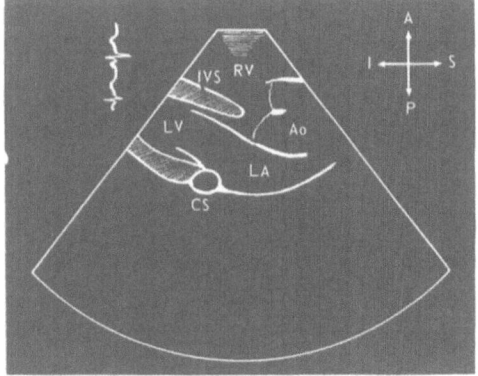

Fig. 6-4 Fallot's tetralogy. diastolic frame showing dilatation of the coronary sinus (CS) due to an associated abnormal systemic venous return (left superior vena cava)

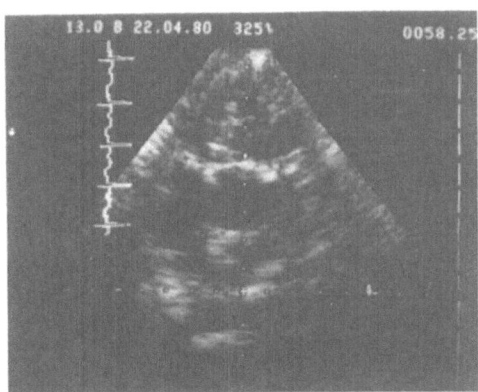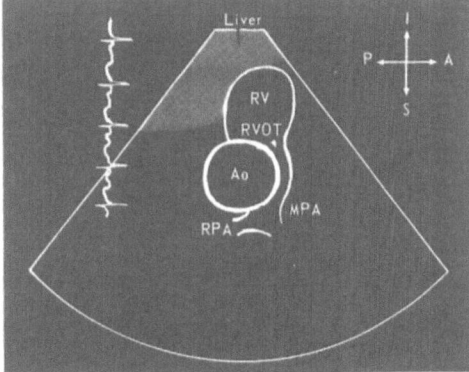

Fig. 6-5 Subcostal view from a patient with Fallot's tetralogy showing stenosis of the infundibulum and main pulmonary artery

— Contrast: At ventricular level, the contrast is first visualised in the right ventricle. During the following diastole, it appears in the left ventricle anterior to the mitral valve, confirming the ventricular septal defect and excluding ASD (Fallot).

At the base, both vessels are opacified simultaneously in systole, without contrast in the left atrium. The main pulmonary artery and its branches are also opacified, giving a better appreciation of any narrowing[180].

C) *Diagnostic pitfalls and comments:*

These recordings are often difficult from a technical point of view because of deformation of the thoracic cage: subcostal views are therefore particularly helpful (fig. 6-5).

The location of the transducer in M mode recordings from the parasternal area is critical: if the transducer is placed too high, an artificial image of overriding aorta may be produced (false positive): on the over hand, if the transducer is in a low position, true overriding may be missed (false negative) (fig. 6-6). Before confirming or excluding the diagnosis of a dextro-position of the basal vessel, repeated scanning should be performed at different levels on the chest and from the subcostal area (see fig. 3-18).

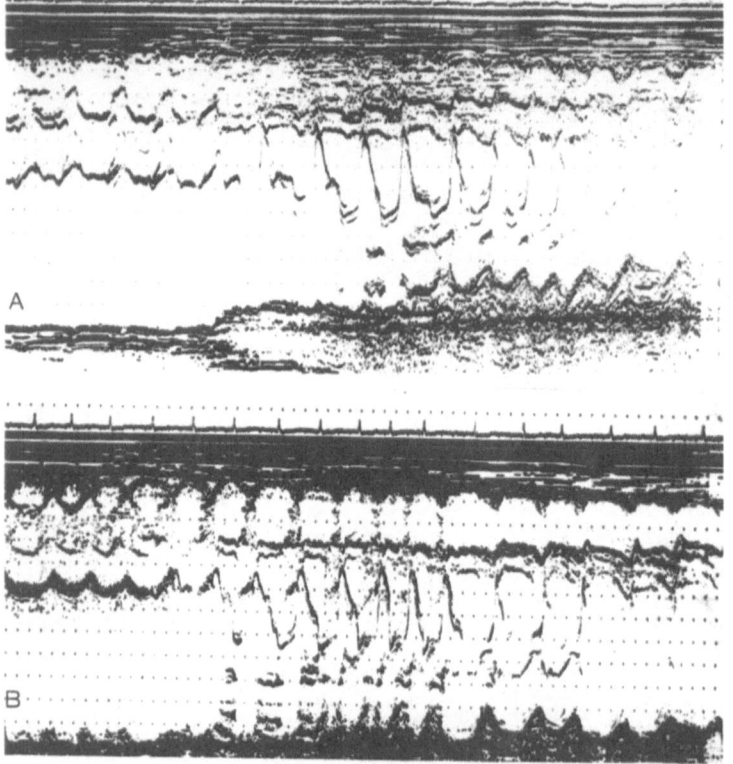

Fig. 6-6

False overriding of the aorta
A- Correct transducer position
B- M mode scan with the transducer at an abnormally high position producing false overriding

Although detection of the pulmonary valve confirms Fallot's tetralogy in this context[29], the inability to record it on M mode does not exclude the diagnosis as it may be very difficult to visualise, due to hypoplasia and its abnormal spatial orientation; in fact, Fallot and truncus arteriosus cannot really be distinguished without 2D echo. Nevertheless, the left atrial dimension in Fallot's tetralogy and "pseudo-truncus", without palliative surgery, is usually small, whilst in common truncus arteriosus it is usually normal[2].

In large VSDs aorto-septal discontinuity may be recorded but there is no dextro-position of the aorta.

In double outlet right ventricle, a similar appearance may be recorded but the striking abnormality is aorto-mitral discontinuity[63] (see next section).

After surgical correction, septal continuity with the systemic artery is normal and the patch may be directly visualised as a dense, passive echo (fig. 6-7, 6-8). Reduction in the RV/LV ratio is usual; when this is not observed, a poor surgical result is to be feared[2] [219] (fig. 6-9).

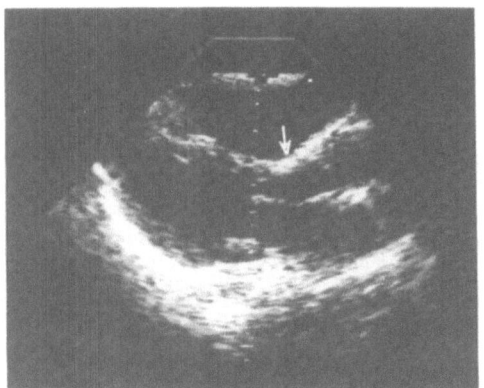 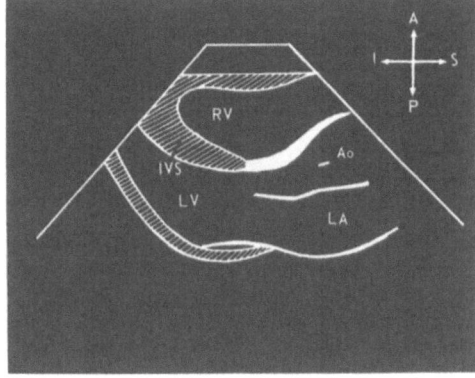

* **Fig. 6-7** Fallot's tetralogy after surgical correction long axis view: diastolic frame showing normal aorto-septal continuity. The patch is arrowed

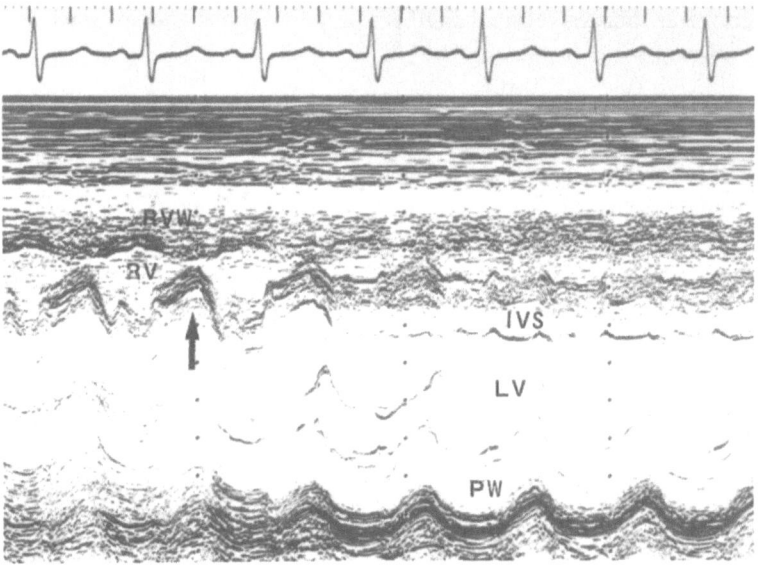

Fig. 6-8
Fallot's tetralogy after surgical correction M mode scan showing the echos reflected by the patch which has a passive motion and which is in continuity with the IVS

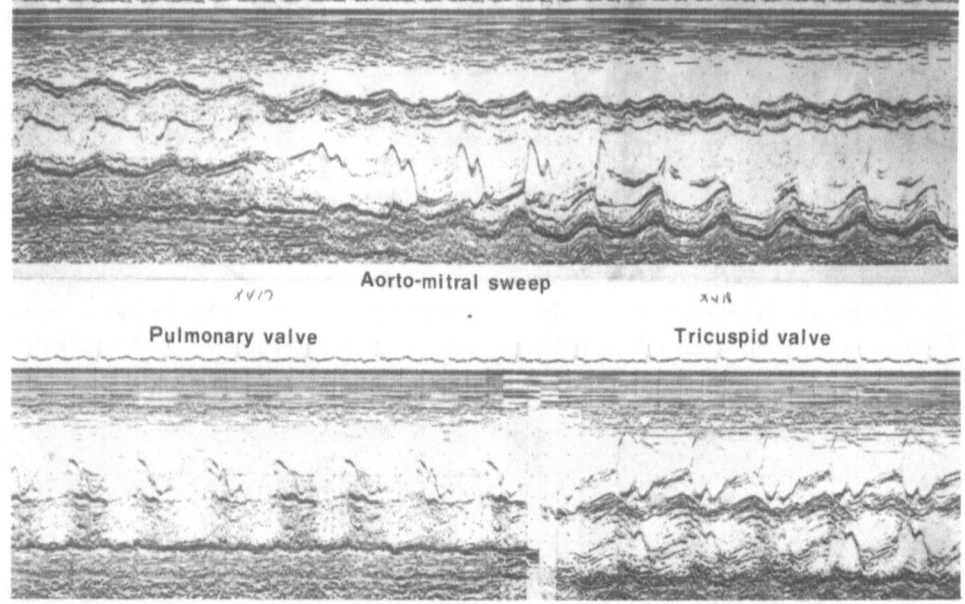

Fig. 6-9 Fallot's tetralogy: postoperative M mode echocardiogram showing normal aorto-septal continuity on the scan and **persistant** premature opening of the pulmonary valve on the pulmonary valve echogram

6.2. DOUBLE OUTLET RIGHT VENTRICLE (DORV)

A) *Anatomy*[142]:

This is a complex cyanotic lesion; the two great arteries, each with its own persistent conus, come off the anatomical right ventricle. This leads to discontinuity between the left atrioventricular valve and the orifices of the two great arteries which are all located at the same level.

A high subpulmonary VSD is associated when both great arteries are in the same anatomical plane, with the pulmonary artery on the left (Taussig - Bing), or when the aorta is anterior and the pulmonary artery to the left (transposition of the great arteries). The VSD is located in the subaortic region when the antero posterior relationship of the arteries is preserved: this is the commonest form, and it may be confused with Fallot's tetralogy.

(fig. 6-10)

B) *Diagnostic signs:*

In all forms, two ventricular chambers are distinguished, the anteriorly positioned one being dilated. Two great arteries are recorded, the more posterior one overriding the septum. The principal finding is a discontinuity between the posterior vessel and the posterior atrioventricular valve, separated by a mass of echos representing the conus[27][240] (fig. 6-11).

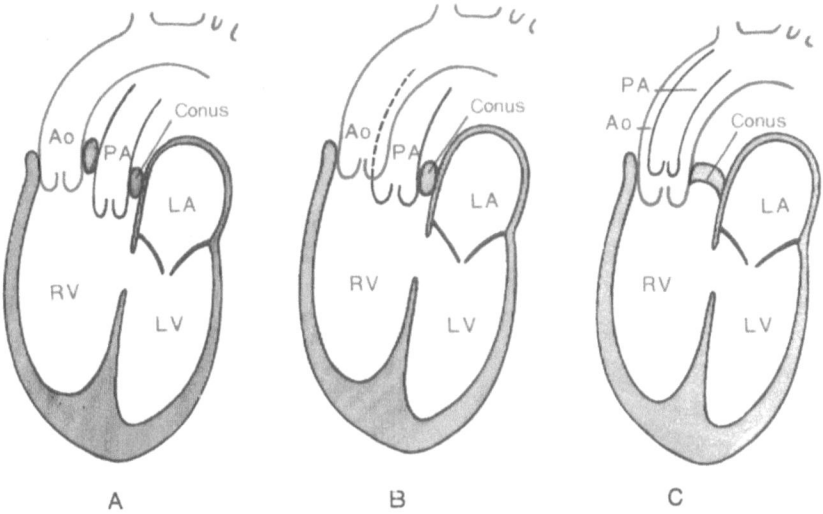

Fig. 6-10 Double outlet right ventricle anatomic typer
A- TAUSSING-BING type
B- Transposed type
C- Pseudo-Fallot type

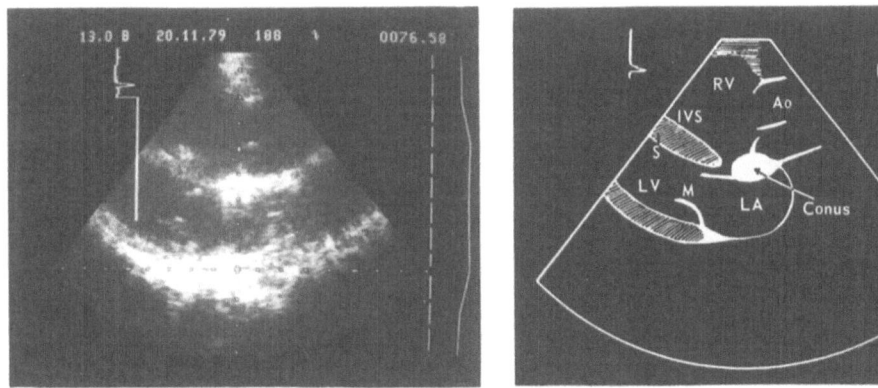

Fig. 6-11 2D long axis view of a patient with double outlet right ventricle.
A"pseudo-Fallot" form; the conus (✐) is the dense mass of echos
causing discontinuity between the mitral valve echos and the aorta

In 2D, the common right ventricular origin of both arteries is particularly well seen in long axis views (fig. 6-12).

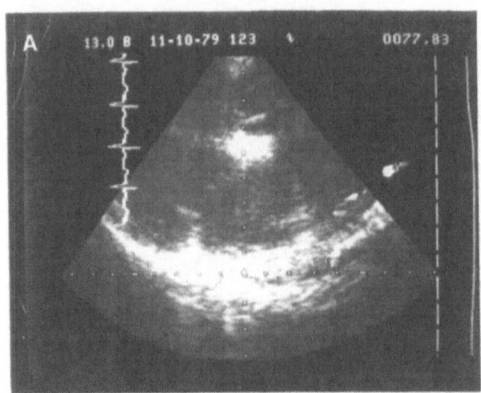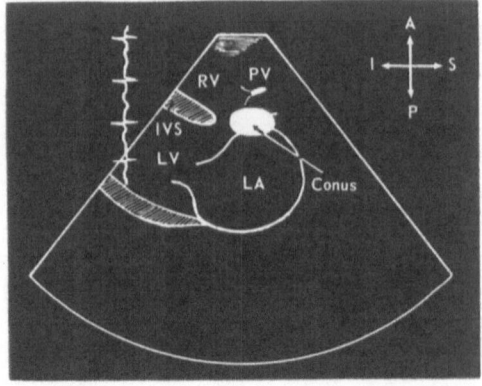

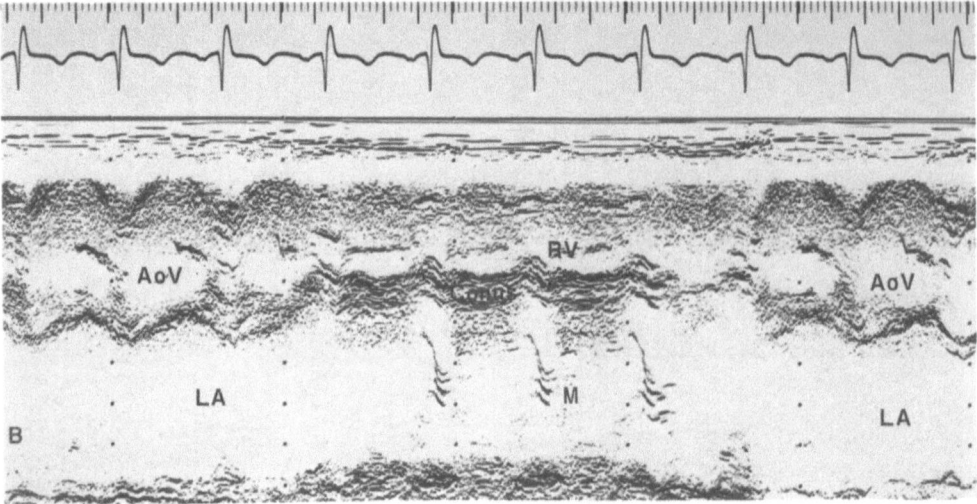

Fig. 6 -12

A- 2D long axis view: double outlet right ventricle of the Taussig-Bing variety showing discontinuity between the pulmonary and mitral valves due to the subpulmonary conus

B- M mode scan from the same patient showing discontinuity between the mitral and aortic echos due to the subaortic conus

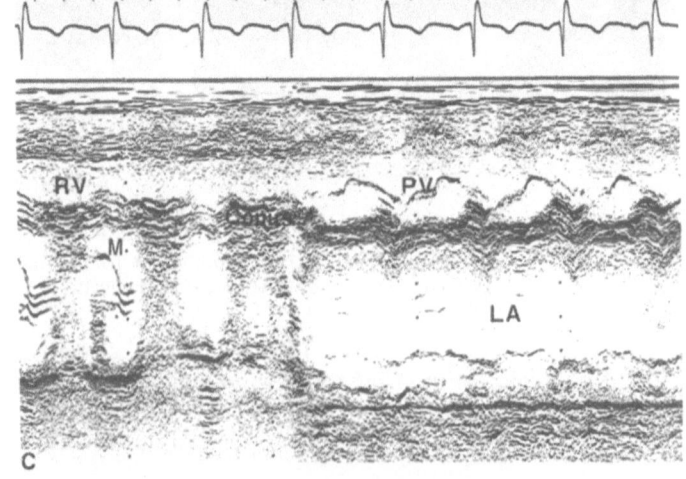

C- M mode scanning from the mitral valve and the second great vessel identified as the pulmonary artery by studying the systolic time intervals: a subpulmonary conus is also visualised

On M mode, the diagnosis depends on the demonstration of discontinuity between the mitral valve and the posterior vessel: this is defined as a posterior displacement of at least 1 cm of the systolic mitral echo with respect to the posterior wall of this great artery. However, the separation may be less in neonates.

A false image of discontinuity may also be produced with unusually high transducer positions[27] [63].

In all cases, 2D echo is essential to confirm the diagnosis.

The precise anatomical variety of DORV is difficult to determine as yet, but 2D echo, with contrast studies, may help solve this problem in the future.

The principal differential diagnosis remains Fallot's tetralogy.

6.3. TRANSPOSITION OF THE GREAT ARTERIES

6.3.1. D transposition

A) *Anatomy:*

This is the classical form of the anomaly. Rotation of the embryological cardiac tube occurs normally to the right so that the ventricles and atria are in their normal positions. However, the position of the great arteries is inverted, the pulmonary artery arising from the left ventricle and the aorta from the right ventricle. The development of the subaortic conus is the factor responsible for the abnormal, anterior, superior and rightward malposition of the aorta. The pulmonary artery is in continuity with the mitral valve and located to the left, posteriorly and inferiorly[142] [217].

This results in two circulations in parallel with venous, desatured blood entering the systemic circulation via the aorta, a situation incompatible with life unless mixing with oxygenated blood occurs at atrial, ventricular or ductal levels. Other malformations may be associated, the most common being valvular and infundibular pulmonary stenosis (40 % cases) Nadas[142].

B) *Diagnostic signs:*

M mode examination necessitates slow scanning from the great arteries to the ventricles, in order to determine the spatial orientation of the great vessels and their continuity with the ventricles, and rapid recording of the two semilunar valves in the great arteries in order to measure the systolic time intervals (a good ECG tracing is essential).

Classically (fig. 6-13), one great artery (aorta) is located anteriorly and to the right, and the other (pulmonary artery) posteriorly and to the left[78]. The earlier closure of the valve in the anteriorly situated vessel identifies it as the aorta. Hirschfield[91] measured the systolic time intervals and showed an increased LVET/RVET ratio (1,22 for normal values of 0,80) and a decreased ratio of the preejection periods[192]. Milner[138] suggested that inversion of the mitral/tricuspid closure relationship was a good sign of transposition (tricuspid closure before mitral closure).

The two great arteries are often recorded simultaneously[40] but this sign is not specific as the same appearance is sometines observed in neonates (fig. 6-13).

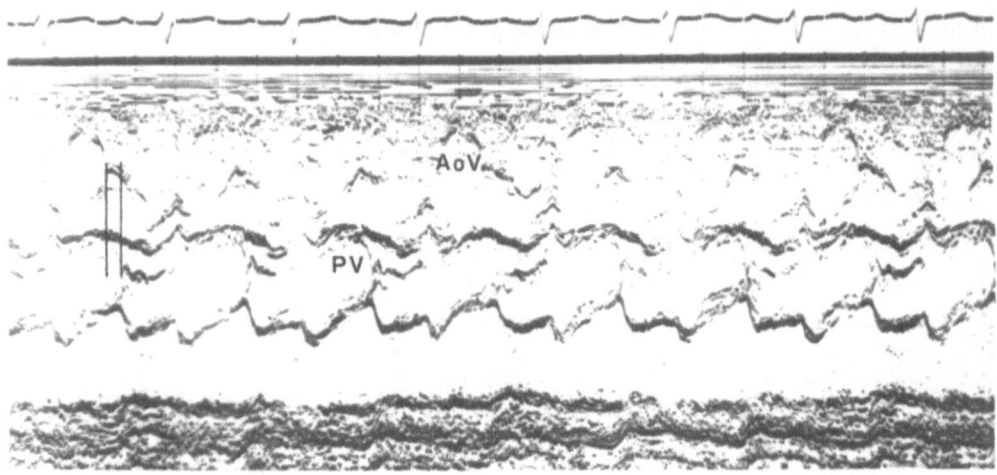

Fig. 6-13 D transposition: the valve of the anterior great vessel closes before that of the posterior vessel. The anterior vessel is therefore the aorta, and the posterior the pulmonary artery

Particular attention must be given to scanning the left ventricular outflow tract in order to detect subvalvular pulmonary stenosis or a large VSD[147] [235] (fig. 6-14).

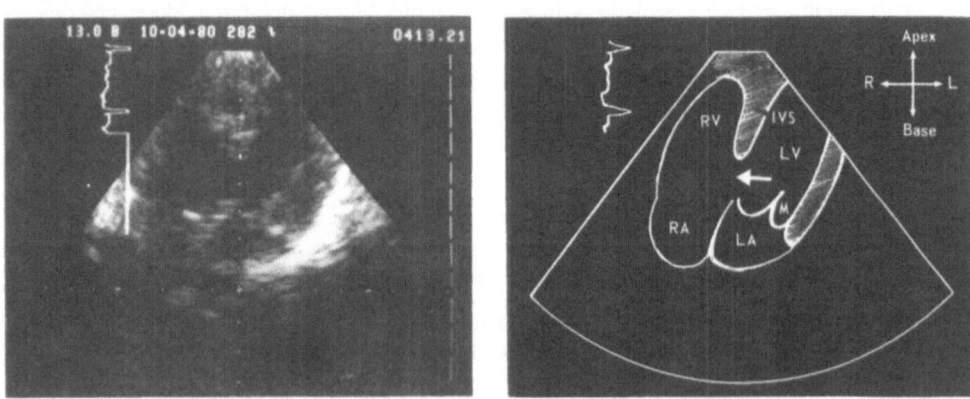

Fig. 6-14 D-Transposition. The visualisation of the associated VSD (✗). In addition, mitral valve prolapse involving both leaflets may be observed

2D: The diagnosis is easier as the spatial orientation of the great arteries may be directly visualised. The two most useful incidences are:

— the short axis view of the base of the heart, which shows two parallel great arteries, the aorta anteriorly and the pulmonary artery behind[88] [103] [170] (fig. 6-15);

— the long axis view from the subcostal position shows the main pulmonary artery and its bifurcation coming off the left ventricle, so confirming the diagnosis[11].

Contrast studies: Their main use is more in the detection of associated malformations (shunts) than in the diagnosis of transposition itself.

C) *Diagnostic pitfalls and comments:*

Apart from cases with associated complex malformations, the 2D diagnosis of D-transposition is relatively easy. The main problems are encountered in M mode as it is very difficult to determine the orientation of the great arteries especially in the neonate, when the aorta and pulmonary artery are often recorded simultaneously. Also, when the pulmonary vascular resistances are high, the systolic ejection times may be similar[83]:

• DORV with transposition gives rise to the same abnormal relationship of the great arteries, but the discontinuity between the posterior vessel and the mitral valve remains.

• After operation (Mustard's procedure) the baffle (vena cava - mitral valve) may be recorded as a linear echo within the left atrium on M mode echo[111]. Diastolic mitral, and occasionally tricuspid fluttering is usually observed[3].

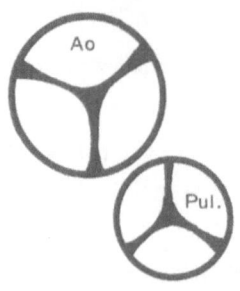

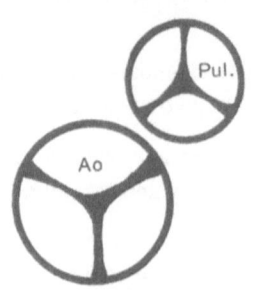

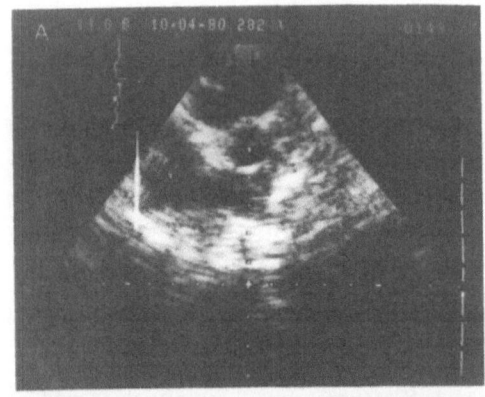

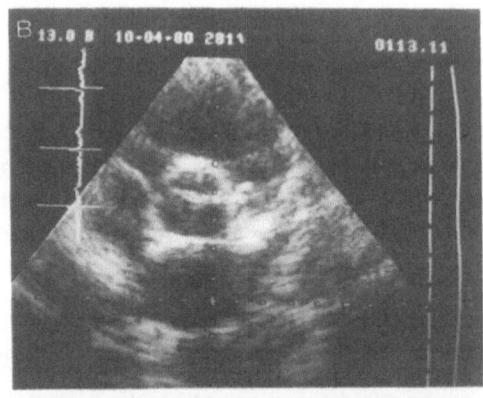

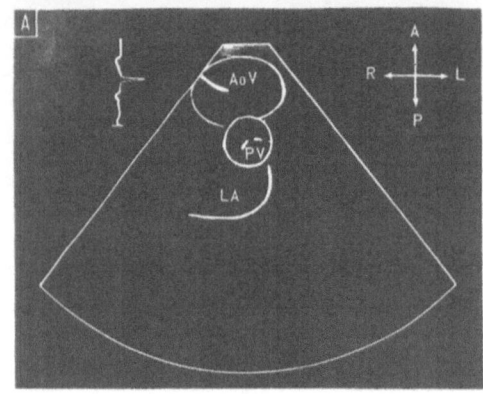

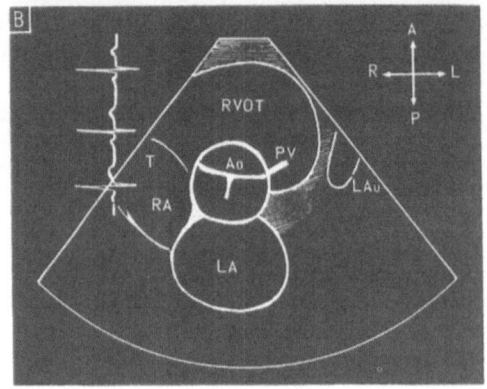

D-Transpo   Normal

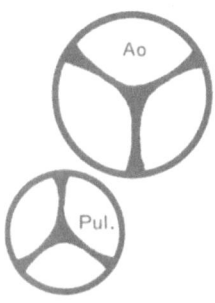

Fig. 6-15

The relative positions of the great vessels
in D-Transposition, in the normal subject
and in L-Transposition

A- The aorta is anterior and to the right
and the pulmonary artery posteriorly
and to the left

B- The aorta is posterior, the pulmonary
artery anterior and to left, with its
infundibulum curving around the aorta

C- The aorta is anterior and to the left,
and the pulmonary artery posteriorly
and to the right

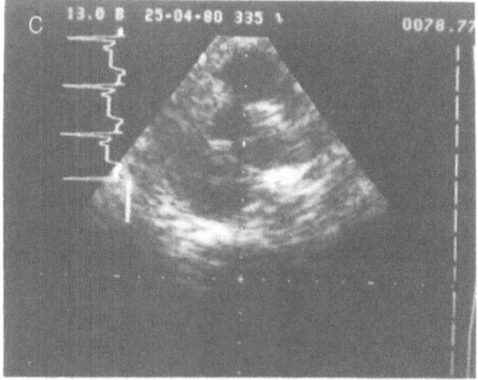

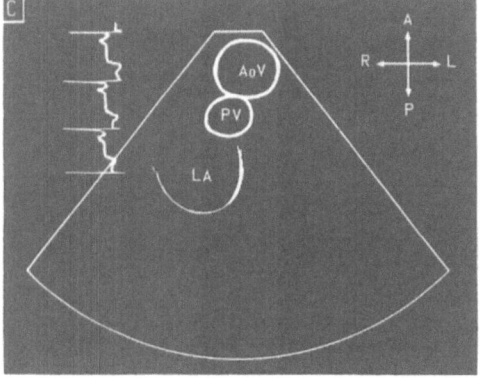

L-Transpo

- The 2D echo visualises the baffle between the two atria on apical, 4-chamber views (fig. 6-16).

The injection of contrast helps determine the patency of the baffle and detects any associated regurgitation (fig. 6-17).

Finally, RV function under systemic pressures may also be analysed.

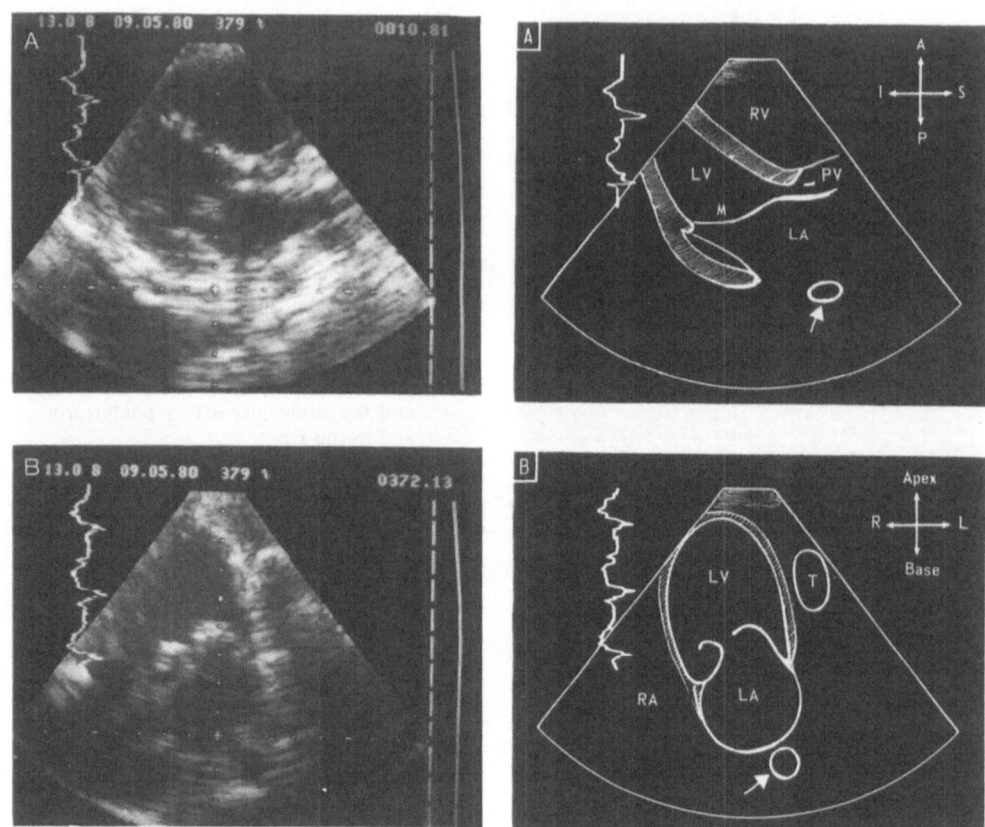

Fig. 6-16 Postoperative echocardiogram of the same patient as fig. 6-15
A- The VDS has been corrected but there is some residual infundibular stenosis. The arrowed circular echo behind the left atrium corresponds to the baffle in front of the pulmonary veins (Sennig's operation)
B- Apical view. The baffle in atrium is seen (✔). Near the lateral LV wall, the Ionescu tube is seen (from the apex to pulmonary artery)

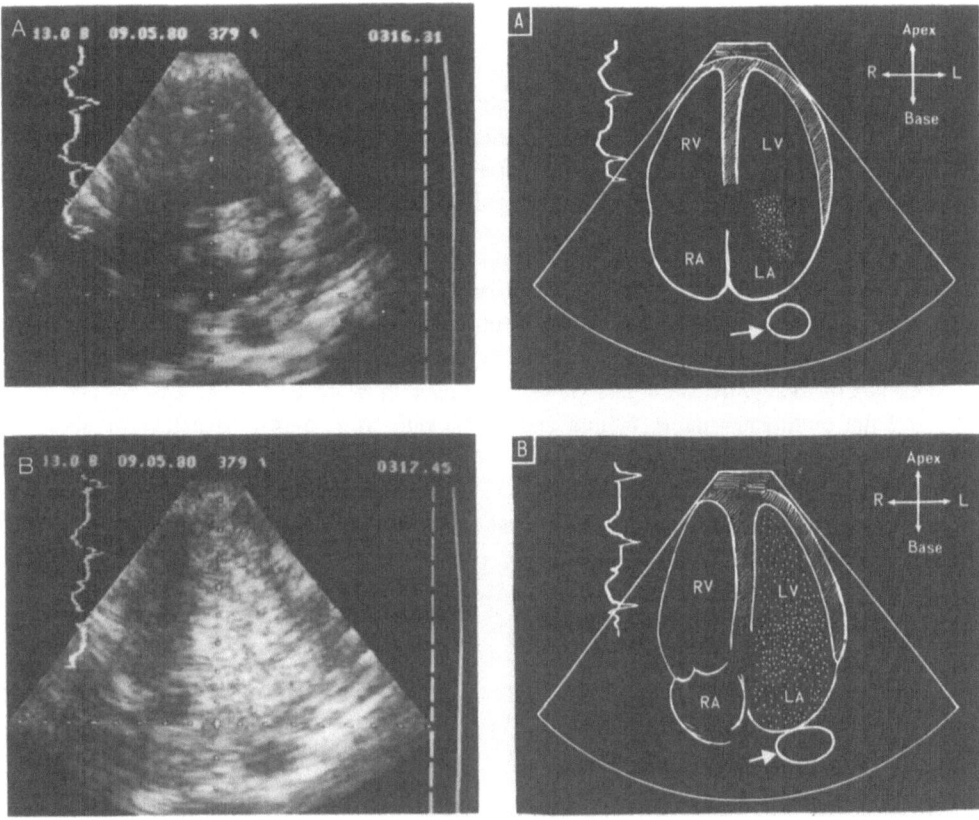

Fig. 6-17 Contrast studies in the same patient as fig. 6-16
A- Opacification of the left atrium above the mitral valve
B- Opacification of the left ventricle with no apparent
     left-to-right shunt

6.3.2. L-Transposition or Corrected Transposition of the Great Arteries

A) *Anatomy*

The primitive cardiac tube rotates to the left so that the morphological right ventricle is located on the left side: the two ventricles (ventricular inversion)[215], situated side by side, lose their normal antero-posterior relationship, the septum being in the saggital plane. The aorta, situated on the left and anteriorly (presence of a subaortic conus), arises from the right ventricle. The pulmonary artery is posterior and on the right, and arises from the left ventricle. If there is an anatomical transposition, the systemic and pulmonary circuits are in series, and from a physiological point of view, the circulation may be considered as normal; however, the right ventricle and the tricuspid valve are subject to a regime of systemic pressures.

Associated malformations are extremely common (59 out of 60 cases in Nadas' series)[142]; the most common are VSD, Ebstein's anomaly and obstructions to ventricular ejection.

— *M mode:* The examination is technically very difficult and the left lateral position is useful for recording the septum in its abnormal saggital plane[28] [136]. There are no specific signs on M mode; discontinuity between the tricuspid valve and the aorta due to the conus may be recorded with an abnormal orientation of the great arteries, the pulmonary artery being located posteriorly and to the right[193]. These diagnostic problems are easier to resolve with 2D echo.

— *2D*[57] [85] [170]: The ventricle on the left side may be seen to be abnormally trabeculated, suggesting a right ventricle and its atrioventricular valve has three leaflets and multiple papillary muscles (fig. 6-19). The long axis view shows tricuspido-aortic discontinuity due to the presence of the conus; short axis views at the base show the aorta to be anterior and to the left, and the pulmonary artery behind and to the right (fig. 6-14). Apical views show the insertion of the septal leaflet of the left-sided atrioventricular valve to be abnormally low, so identifying it as the tricuspid valve (fig. 6-18) (extreme malposition of its insertion suggests the presence of Ebstein's anomaly). Subcostal views show the pulmonary artery arising from the left ventricle without an infundibulum (fig. 6-20A).

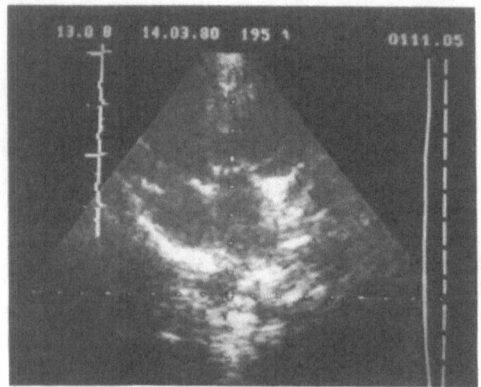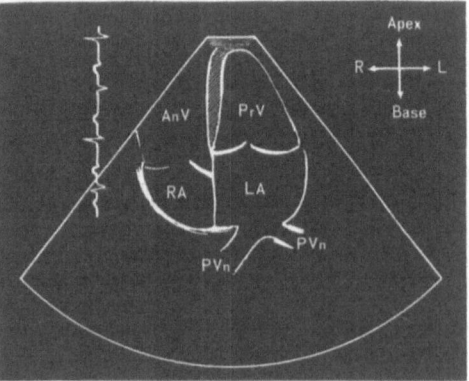

Fig. 6-18   L-Transposition: 4 chamber apical view.
The atrioventricular valve of the posterior ventricle (PV) is inserted nearer to the apex than the atrioventricular valve of the anterior ventricle (AV). The pulmonary veins (PVn) drain normally into the left atrium

AnV: anterior ventricle
PrV: posterior ventricle
PVn: pulmonic vein

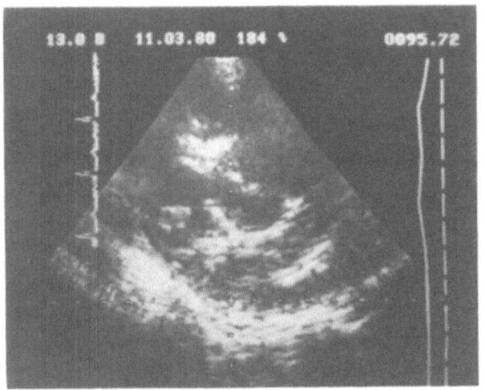 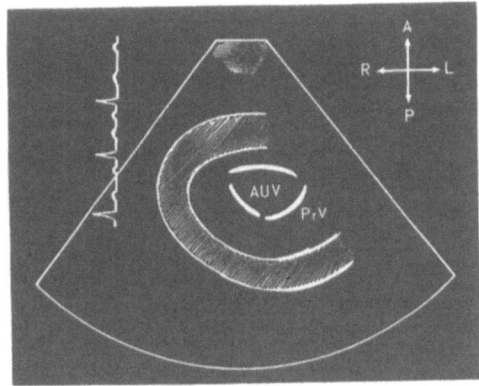

Fig. 6-19 L-Transposition of the great arteries: 2D short axis view of the posterior ventricle (PV). The atrioventricular valve has three leaflets which identifies it as the tricuspid valve

PrV: posterior ventricle   AVV: auriculo-ventricular valve

Contrast: The morphology of the heart chambers and associated shunts may be demonstrated (fig. 6-20).

C) *Diagnostic pitfalls and comments:*

The problems occur in the interpretation of the M mode echo which may appear to be normal, suggestive of an endocardial cushion defect due to the abnormal insertion of the left-sided atrioventricular valve or double outlet right ventricle due to the subaortic conus. 2D echo will correct the diagnosis.

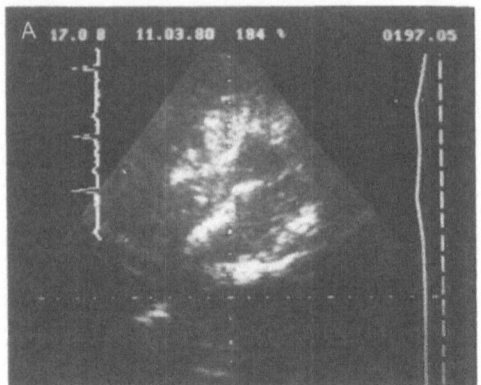
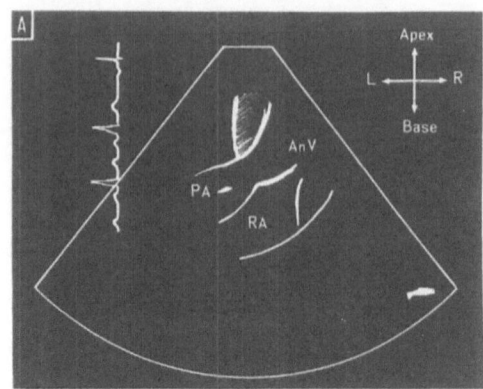
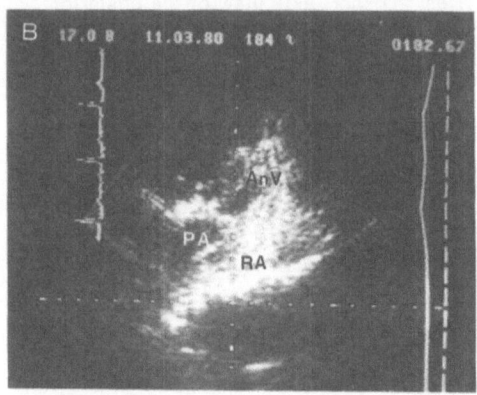
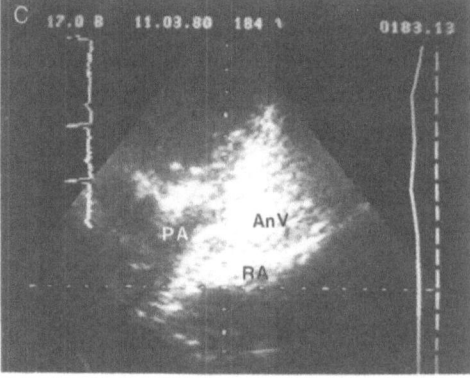
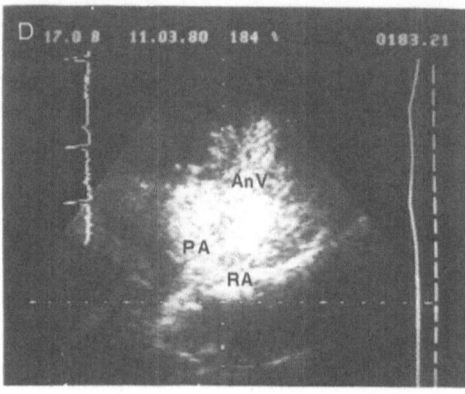

Fig. 6-20 A- L-Transposition: the anterior chamber (anatomical left ventricle)
leads directly on to the pulmonary artery without on intermediary
pulmonary infundibulum

B- Contrast study: the right atrium is the first chamber to be opacified.
The contrast then flows into the anterior chamber (fig. C) and then
into the pulmonary artery (fig. D)

CHAPTER 7

OTHERS MALFORMATIONS

7.1. SINGLE VENTRICLE (Common Ventricle)

A) *Anatomy:*

In this anomaly, a single ventricle (absent interventricular septum) receives blood crossing two separate or a single common atrioventricular valve. In the commonest form the infundibulum is situated anteriorly on the left or right side according to the rotation of the primitive cardiac tube. The relationship of the great arteries may be normal, or D-, or L-transposition may be present[142] [214]

B) *Diagnostic signs:*

— *M mode:* The diagnosis is confirmed when the following appearances are observed[26] [135] [136]:

• simultaneous recording of two atrioventricular valves without intervening septal echos (fig. 7-1);

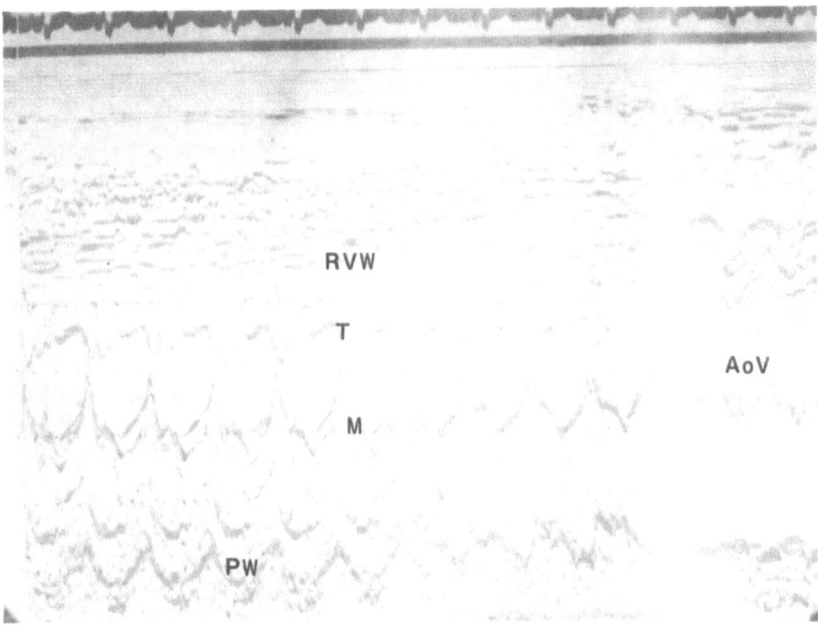

Fig. 7-1 Single or common ventricle
M mode scan showing complete absence of septal echos between the tricuspid and mitral valves which are recorded simultaneously

• a small anterior chamber without an atrioventricular valve[55] [183] [184] (fig. 7-2);

• usually, the posterior atrioventricular valve is in continuity with a great vessel.

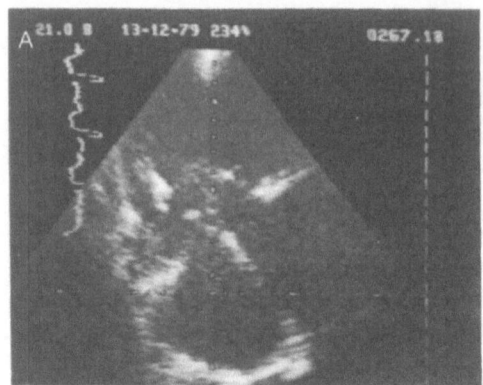
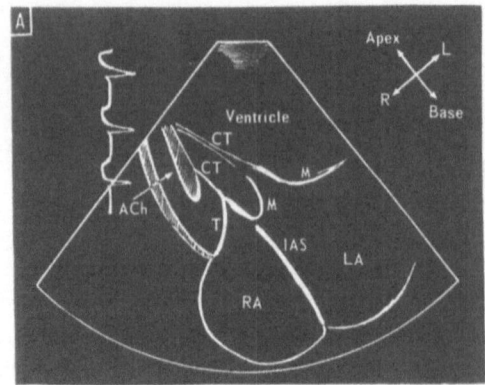

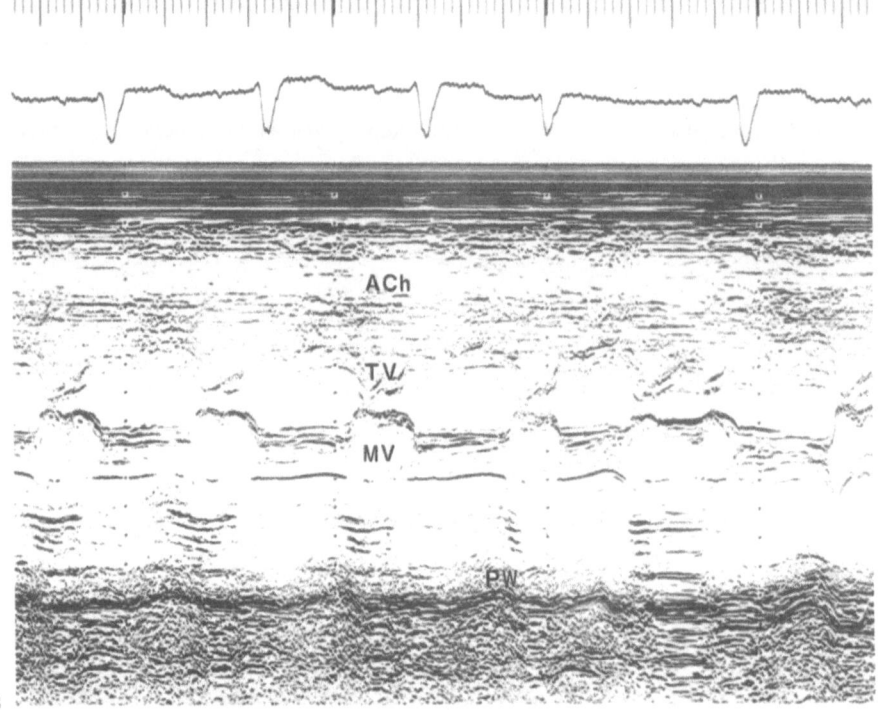

In cases with single atrioventricular valve, the anterior chamber is not usually present: this valve has a large amplitude and occupies the whole ventricular cavity without septal interposition. In transposition of the great arteries, the previously described anatomical changes are found.

— 2D: This confirms total absence of an interventricular septum (especially with contrast injection), defines the position of the great arteries, the number of atrioventricular valves and the presence of an accessory outflow tract[188] (fig. 7-2). In forms with a single atrioventricular valve, the interatrial septum is often absent[183].

132

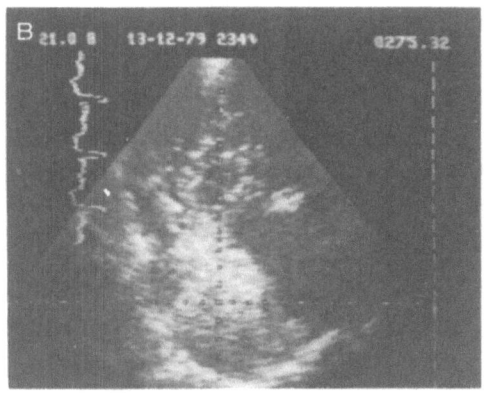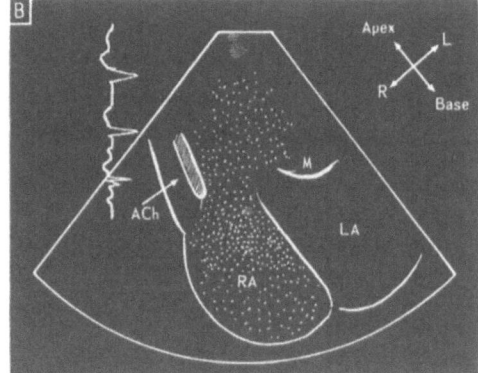

Fig. 7-2 Single ventricle

    A- 2D: showing two atrioventricular valves without an interventricular
       septum. The chordae (CT) seem to converge on the anterior
       ventricular wall. The residual hypoplastic anterior chamber (ACh)
       is clearly visible (✗)

    B- Contrast study: the left atrium and the anterior chamber are the
       only non-opacified chambers

    C- M mode: echocardiogram showing the two atrioventricular valves
       without intervening septal echos. The residual hypoplastic
       anterior chamber is visualised anteriorly
       ACh: anterior chamber

C) Diagnostic pitfalls and comments:

Multiple M mode scans of the ventricle are required to be sure that the interventricular septum is absent, as endocardial cushion defects and overriding tricuspid valves can give the same appearances in the routine position. Extreme forms of endocardial cushion defect are, in fact, variants of single ventricle (in cases with single atrioventricular valve): the only distinguishing feature is the presence of an accessory outflow tract.

In cases of tricuspid atresia and right ventricular hypoplasia, 2D contrast studies orientate the diagnosis by demonstrating the consecutive opacification of the right atrium, left atrium (via ASD) and the left ventricle. In left ventricular hypoplasia, the accessory chamber is situated posteriorly, whilst it is always anterior in single ventricle.

After surgery, the dense, non-contractile echo of the patch between the two ventricular cavities, each with its own valve, may be observed[183].

7.2. OVERRIDING TRICUSPID VALVE

A) Anatomy:

The tricuspid valve is abnormally placed, and the right atrium partially or totally empties into the left ventricle through an VSD of endocardial cushion type with resulting right ventricular hypoplasia.

133

B) *Diagnostic signs*

The two atrioventricular valves are recorded simultaneously without invervening septal echos at the base of the heart. Scanning down towards the apex shows the septal leaflet of the tricuspid valve to be posterior to the left septal side in diastole. The right ventricular cavity is small[112] [181] (fig. 7-3).

C) *Diagnostic pitfalls and comments*

Endocardial cushion defects may give similar appearances but the right ventricle is usually of normal size.

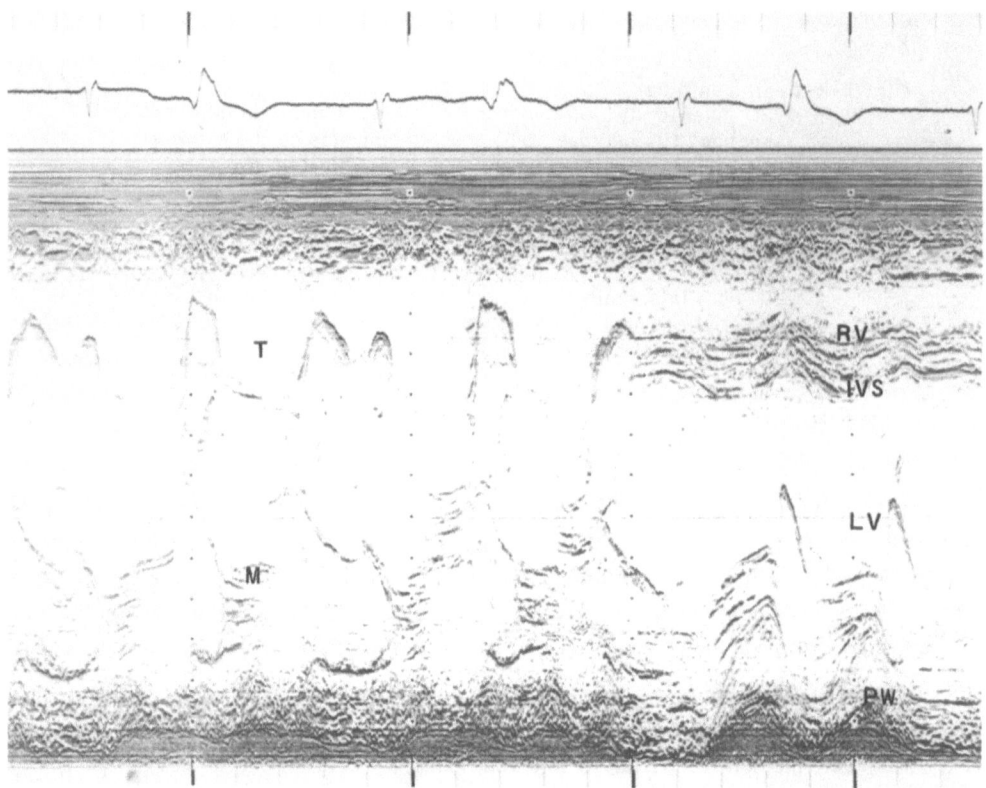

Fig. 7-3 Overriding tricuspid valve: the septal tricuspid leaflet is posterior to the interventricular septum and lies in the LV

CHAPTER 8

A SEGMENTAL APPROACH TO THE DIAGNOSIS OF CONGENITAL HEART DISEASE

The diagnostic signs of each anomaly have been described in the preceding chapters, but some have similar echocardiographic appearances. A logical approach, step by step, leads to a general appreciation of the various malformations which may be present and a clearly deduced diagnosis.

A segmental approach, as suggested by Van Praagh[213] [214] [215] [216] [217] determining the relative position and relationships of the atria, ventricles and great arteries makes possible precise diagnosis by echocardiography[57] [126] [193].

8.1. ATRIAL SITUS

The position of the right atrium depends on that of the abdominal viscera and the lungs. The inferior vena cava which is in the same side, is an easy landmark in 2D echo[57] [126]. The presence of an interatrial septum is determined and the respective sizes of the two atria assessed[10].

8.2. VENTRICULAR SITUS

There is no dissociation between the atrioventricular valves and their respective ventricles. The tricuspid valve is always in the anatomical right ventricle. Therefore, the identification of these valves defines the ventricles. This step is often difficult with M mode alone. 2D echo[57] [85], however, gives an immediate diagnosis on the following signs:

— the tricuspid ring is inserted nearer the apex;

— the appearance of the valvular orifices on short axis views (oval, "fish's-mouth" appearance of the mitral valve, the three leaflets of the tricuspid valve);

— the two papillary muscles in the anatomical left ventricle and the more trabeculated appearance of the right.

The suggested M mode criteria (continuity of the posterior AV valve with semi-lunar cusp to identify the mitral valve[135] [193], and delay in tricuspid valve closure[126] appear to be less specific.

The visualisation of a tricuspid valve to the right and anteriorly confirms normal rotation of the primitive cardiac tube (D-rotation). The presence of an interventricular septum excludes single (or common) ventricle, and its position enables assessment of the size of the respective ventricles.

8.3. IDENTIFICATION OF THE GREAT ARTERIES

The use of systolic time intervals with M mode echo helps identify the great arteries, the pulmonary being longer than the aortic ejection period[91] in the absence of pulmonary hypertension, which is common in the neonatal period. When the valves have been identified, the orientation and relationship of the great arteries must be defined: normally, the aorta is posterior and to the right and the pulmonary artery anterior and to the left. If the great artery on the right is also anterior, D-transposition should be suspected[40] [78]. In addition, the origin of the pulmonary artery is wider (in the absence of pulmonary stenosis)[212] than that of the systemic artery, but this may be difficult to assess.

The presence of two great vessels may be confirmed on 2D echo, a fact which is often difficult with M mode alone (differentiation between Fallot's tetralogy and truncus arteriosus[29]). In short axis views of the base of the heart, which are often easier to perform from the subcostal area, the infundibulum normally curves anterior to the aorta which is situated posteriorly and to the right. It may be followed out to the main pulmonary artery and its branching into the left and right pulmonary arteries. The posteriorly situated vessel may be followed to its arch, which is visible from the suprasternal[172] [232] [81] and subcostal areas[11].

8.4. VENTRICULO-ARTERIAL CONTINUITY

The subvalvular conus is normally always situated anteriorly, resulting in tricuspid pulmonary discontinuity and mitro aortic continuity. Mitro-aortic discontinuity[27] is suggestive of either L-transposition or DORV. The relationship of each great artery to the septum defines their relationship with the ventricles. Dextroposition of the aorta in Fallot's tetralogy, anterior origin of the two great vessels in DORV.

8.5. DETECTION OF SHUNTS

They may either be diagnosed directly by the visualisation of septal discontinuity, or indirectly by the recording of signs of atrioventricular volume overload, or by using contrast technique.

A precise diagnosis and an assessment of the severity of congenital malformations is facilitated by this complete segmental approach, integrating the clinical, ECG and X-Ray findings.

APPENDIX

Normal values oι ιne principal echocardiographic measures. (Echocardiographic laboratory Institut de Cardiologie de Quebec 44 adults)

Table I: Normal values in adults (mean ± standard deviation)

B.S.A. (m²)	1.70 ± .10
Dd (mm)	46.3 ± 4.38
DS (mm)	29.6 ± 3.57
RV (mm)	13.6 ± 2.61
LA (mm)	28.9 ± 3.32
Ao (mm)	27.2 ± 3.96
VM g	163.8 ± 46.0
EF. M. slope (mm/s)	157 ± 40.6
RV/LV	.297 ± .056
LA/Ao	1.050 ± .168
S/P.W.	1.02 ± .75
V.C.F. (circ/s)	1.18 ± .238
H/R	.360 ± .042
%Dd	36.03 ± 5.44

Table II: Normal values of ventricular walls in adults (mean ± standard deviation)

Posterior wall:

Twd (mm)	8.35 ± 1.03
Tws (mm)	13.48 ± 1.53
CT (s)	.358 ± .30
%Tw	62.4 ± 15.8
VTwC (tw. u/s)	1.75 ± .444

Interventricular septum

Twd (mm)	8.5 ± 1.03
Tws (mm)	12.53 ± 1.39
TC (s)	.289 ± .026
%E	47.9 ± 10.5
V. Tw C (tw. u/s)	1.67 ± .413

Table III: Published Normal values: neonates and children (mean and range)

	Nb	Weight kg	BSA m²	RVD (d) mm	LVID d mm	PLVW (twd) mm
Hagan et al	200	3.3 (2.7 - 4.6)	—	11.4 (6.1 - 15)	18.7 (12 - 23.3)	2.6 (1.6 - 3.7)
Meyer et al [136]	50	3.2 (1.9 - 4.3)	—	13 (10 - 17)	16 (12 - 20)	—
Solinger et al [191]	21	2.27	—	12.5 (10.4 - 14.6)	18.9 (16.1 - 21.7)	2.7 (2 - 3.4)
	28	2.73	—	13.1 (11 - 15.2)	19.3 (16.5 - 22.1)	3 (2.3 - 3.7)
	25	3.18	—	13.7 (11.6 - 15.8)	19.8 (17 - 22.6)	3.2 (2.5 - 3.9)
	22	3.64	—	14.4 (12.3 - 16.5)	20.3 (17.5 - 23.1)	3.5 (2.8 - 4.2)
	23	4.09	—	15 (12.9 - 17.11)	20.8 (18 - 23.6)	3.7 (3 - 4.4)
Feigenbaum [54]	24	—	0.5 <	8 (3 - 13)	24 (13 - 22)	5 (4 - 6)
	39	—	0.6 - 1	10 (4 - 18)	34 (24 - 42)	6 (5 - 7)
	29	—	1.. - 1.5	12 (7 - 17)	40 (33 - 47)	7 (6 - 8)

Hagan et al : Hagan A.D., Decley W.J., Sahn D.S. et al : Echocardiographic criteria for normal newborn infants. Circulation 48:1221,1973.

BIBLIOGRAPHY

1. ASSAD-MORELL J.L., TAJIK A.J., GUILIANI E.R.: Echocardiographic analysis of the ventricular septrum, *Progr. Cardiovasc. Dis.*, **17**:219, 1974.

2. ASSAD-MOREL J.L., SEWARD J.B., TAJIK A.J. et al: Echo-Phonocardiographic and contrast studies in conditions associated with systemic arterial trunk overriding the ventricular septum: Truncus arteriosus, tetralogy of Fallot, and pulmonary atresia with ventricular septal defect, *Circulation*, **53**:663, 1976.

3. AZIZ K.U., PAUL M.H., MUSTER A.J.: Echocardiographic localization of interatrial baffle after Mustard operation for dextro transposition of the great arteries, *Am. J. Cardiol.*, **38**:67, 1976.

4. BAKER D.W.: Physical and technical principles in KING D.L., Editor, Diagnostic Ultrasound. *CV Mosby, Saint-Louis,* 1974.

5. BASS J.L. EINZIG S., HONG C.Y. et al: Echocardiographic screnning to assess the severity of congenital aortic stenosis in children, *Am. J. Cardiol.*, **44**:82, 1979.

6. BASS J.L., BEN-SHACHAR G., EDWARDS J.E.: Comparison of M Mode echocardiography and pathologic findings in the hypoplastic left heart syndrome, *Am. J. Cardiol.*, **45**:79, 1980.

7. BELENKIE I., NUTTER D.O., CLARK D.W. et al: Assessment of left ventricular dimensions and function by echocardiography, *Am. J. Cardiol.*, **31**:755, 1973.

8. BERRY T.E., AZIZ K.U., PAUL M.H.: Echocardiographic assessment of discrete subaortic stenosis in childhood, *Am. J. Cardiol.*, **43**:957, 1979.

9. BETRIU A., WIGEL E.D., FELDERHOFF C.H. et al: Prolapse of the mitral valve associated with secundum atrial septal defect, *Am. J. Cardiol.*, **35**:363, 1975.

10. BIERMAN F.Z., WILLIAMS R.G.: Subxiphoid two dimensional imaging of the interatrial septum in infant and neonates with congenital heart disease, *Circulation*, **60**:80, 1979.

11. BIERMAN F.Z., WILLIAMS R.G.: Prospective diagnosis of D Transposition of the great arteires in neonates by subxiphoid two dimensional echocardiography, *Circulation*, **60**:1496, 1979.

12. BOM N., LANCEE C.T., VAN ZWIETEN G., KLOSTER F.E. et al: Multiscan echocardiography. I. Technical description, *Circulation*, **48**:1066, 1973.

13. BOMMER W., WEINERT L., NEUMANN A. et al: Determination of right atrial size and right ventricular size by two dimensionnal echocardiography, *Circulation*, **60**:91, 1979.

14. BOUGHNER D.R., PERSAUD J.A.: Parachute mitral valve: echocardiographic findings resembling idiopathic hypertrophic subaortic stenosis, *J. Clin. Ultrasound*, **4**:213, 1976.

15. BURGGRAF G.W., CRAIGE E.: Echocardiographic studies of left ventricular wall motion and dimensions after valvular heart surgery, *Am. J. Cardiol.*, **35**:473, 1975.

16. CALDWELL R.L., WEYMAN A.E., HURWITZ R.A. et al: Right ventricular outflow tract assessment by cross-sectional echocardiography in tetralogy of Fallot, *Circulation*, **59**:395, 1979.

17. CALDWELL R.L., WEYMAN A.E., HURWITZ R.A. et al: Cross-sectional echocardiographic evaluation of coronary artery abnormalities in children, *Am. J. Cardiol.*, **45**:467, 1980 (abst).

18. CANALE J.M., SAHN D.J., ALLEN H.D. et al: Factors affecting the real time cross-sectional echocardiographic imaging of ventricular septal defect, *Am. J. Cardiol.*, **45**:467, 1980 (abst).

19. CANEDO M.I., STEFADOUROS M.A., FRANK M.J. et al: Echocardiographic features of cor triatriatum, *Am. J. Cardiol.*, **40**:615, 1977.

20. CARLSEN E.N.: Ultrasound physics for the physician. A brief review, *J. Clin. Ultrasound*, **3**:69, 1975.

21. CARR K.W., ENGLER R.L., FORSYTHE J.R. et al: Measurement of left ventricular ejection fraction by mechanical cross-sectional echocardiography, *Circulation*, **59**:1196, 1979.

22. CHANDRARATNA P.A., BHADURI U., LITTMAN B.B. et al: Echocardiographic findings in persistent truncus arteriosus in a young adult, *Brit. Heart. J.*, **36**:732, 1974.

23. CHAPELLE M., MENSCH B., CABROL C.: Physiopathologie de la valvule mitrale : Etude par ultrasonographie, *Cœur Med. Interne*, **9**:209, 1970.

24. CHANG S., FEIGENBAUM H.: Subxiphoid echocardiography, *J. Clin. Ultrasound*, **1**:14, 1973.

25. CHANG S.: M Mode echocardiographic techniques and pattern recognition, *Lea et Febiger, Philadelphia,* 1976.

26. CHESLER E., JOFFE H.S., VECHT R. et al: Ultrasound cardiography in single ventricle and the hypoplastic left and right heart syndromes, *Circulation*, **42**:123, 1970.

27. CHESLER E., JOFFE H.S., BECK W. et al: Echocardiographic recognition of mitral semi lunar valve discontinuity, *Circulation*, **43**:725, 1971.

28. CHESLER E., JOFFE H.S., BECK W. et al: Echocardiography in the diagnosis of congenital heart disease, *Pediatr. Clin. North. Am.*, **18**:1163, 1971.

29. CHUNG K.J., ALEXON C.G., MANNING J.A. et al: Echocardiography in truncus arteriosus: The value of pulmonic valve detection, *Circulation*, **43**:281, 1973.

30. CHUNG K.J., MANNING J.A., LIPCHIK E.O. et al: Isolated supravalvular stenosing ring of left atrium: diagnosis before operation and successful surgical treatment, *Chest.*, **65**:25, 1974.

31. CLARKE D.R., STARK J., DE LEVAL M. et al: Total anomalous pulmonary venous drainage in infancy, *Br. Heart. J.*, **39**:436, 1977.

32. COOPER R.H., O'ROURKE R.A., KARLINER J.S. et al: Comparison of ultrasound and cineangiographic measurements of the mean rate of circumferential fiber shortening in man, *Circulation*, **46**:914, 1972.

33. CORYA B.C., FEIGENBAUM H., RASMUSSEN S. et al: Anterior left ventricular wall echoes in coronary artery disease. Linear scanning with a single element transducer, *Am. J. Cardiol.*, **34**:652, 1974.

34. CRAIGE E.: On the genesis of heart sounds. Contributions made by echocardiographic studies, *Circulation*, **53**:207, 1976.

35. DAVIS R.H., FEIGENBAUM H., CHANG S. et al: Echocardiographic manifestations of discrete subaortic stenosis, *Am. J. Cardiol.*, **33**:277, 1974.

36. DE MARIA A.N., MILLER R.R., AMSTERDAM E.A. et al: Mitral valve early diastolic closing velocity on echogram: relation to sequential diastolic flow and ventricular compliance, *Am. J. Cardiol.*, **37**:693, 1976.

37. DE MARIA A.N., OLIVER L.E., BORGREN H.G. et al: Apparent reduction of aortic and left heart chamber size in atrial septal defect, *Am. J. Cardiol.*, **42**:545, 1978.

38. DE MARIA A.N., NEUMANN A., SCHUBART P.J. et al: Systematic correlation of cardiac chamber size and ventricular performance determined with echocardiography and alterations in heart rate in normal patients, *Am. J. Cardiol.*, **43**:1, 1979.

39. DIAMOND M.A., DILLON J.C., HAINE C.L. et al: Echocardiographic features of atrial septal defect, *Circulation*, **43**:129, 1971.

40. DILLON J.C., FEIGENBAUM H., KONECKE L.L.et al: Echocardiographic manifestations of D Transposition of the great vessels, *Am. J. Cardiol.*, **32**:74, 1973.

41. DILLON J.C., WEYMAN A.E., FEIGENBAUM H. et al: Cross-sectional echocardiographic examination of the interatrial septum, *Circulation*, **55**:115, 1977.

42. DUMESNIL J.G., LAURENCEAU J.L., LABATUT A.: L'épaississement myocardique, un critère valable pour apprécier la fonction ventriculaire gauche régionale : une étude échocardiographique, *Ann. Cardiol. Angeiol.*, **24**:491, 1975.

43. DUMESNIL J.G., LAURENCEAU J.L.: Echocardiographic analysis of left ventricular wall thickness, *Cardio-vasc. Med.*, **2**:1005, 1977.

44. DUMESNIL J.G., SHOUCRI R.M., LAURENCEAU J.L. et al: A mathematical model of the dynamic geometry of the intact left ventricle and its application to clinical data, *Circulation*, **59**:1024, 1979.

45. DROBINSKI G., BEJEAN-LEBUISSON A., EVANS J.I. et al: Formes atypiques de la maladie d'Ebstein : apports et limites de l'echocardiographie et du catheterisme cardiaque, *Ann. Med. Interne*, **130**:459, 1979.

46. EATON L.W., MAUGHAN L., WEISS J.L. et al: Accurate volume determination in the isolated ejecting canine heart from a limited number of two dimensional echocardiographic cross-sections, *Am. J. Cardiol.*, **45**:470, 1980 (abstract).

47. EDLER I., HERTZ C.H.: Use of ultrasonic reflectoscope for continuous recording of movements of heart wall, *Kung. Fysiograf. Sallsk. Lund. Forhandl*, **24**:40, 1954.

48. EDLER I.: Ultrasound cardiogram in mitral valve disease, *Acta Chir. Scand.*, **11**:230, 1956.

49. EDLER I., GUSTAFSON A., KARLEFORS T. et al: Ultrasound echocardiography, *Acta Med. Scand.*, **170**:(suppl. 370) 67, 1961.

50. ELBL F., SOLINGER R., MINKAS K.: Echocardiographic features of pulmonary atresia type I, *Circulation*, **50**:(suppl. III) 142, 1974.

50 bis. FAROOKI Q.Z., HENRY J.G., GREEN E.W.: Echocardiographic spectrum of the hypoplastic left heart syndrome: a clinico pathologic correlation in 19 newborns, *Am. J. Cardiol*, **38**:337, 1976.

51. FEIGENBAUM H., ZAKY A., NASSER W.K.: Use of ultrasound to measure left ventricular stroke volume, *Circulation*, **35**:1092, 1967.

52. FEIGENBAUM H., STONE J.M. LEE D.A. et al: Identification of ultrasound echoes from the left ventricle by use of intracardiac injection of indocyanine green, *Circulation*, **41**:615, 1970.

53. FEIGENBAUM H.: Editorial. Echocardiographic examination of the left ventricle, *Circulation*, **51**:1, 1975.

54. FEIGENBAUM H.: Echocardiography (2nd Edition), *Lea & Fibiger, Philadelphia*, 1976.

55. FELNER J.L., BREWER D.B., FRANCH R.H.: Echocardiographic manifestation of single ventricle, *Am. J. Cardiol.*, **38**:80, 1976.

56. FIRESTONE F.A.: The supersonic reflectoscope an instrument for inspecting the interior of solid parts by means of sound waves, *J. Acoust. Soc. Amer.*, **17**:287, 1945.

57. FOALE R.A., STEFANINI L., RICKARDS A.F. et al: Two dimensional echocardiographic features of corrected transposition, *Am. J. Cardiol.*, **45**:466, 1980 (abst.)

58. FOLLAND E.D., PARISI A.F., MOYNIHAN P.F. et al: Assessment of left ventricular ejection fraction and volumes by real time, two dimensional echocardiography. A comparison of cineangiographic and radionuclide techniques, *Circulation*, **60**:760, 1979.

59. FORTUIN N.J., HOOD W.P. SHERMAN M.E. et al: Determination of left ventricular volumes by ultrasound, *Circulation*, **44**:575, 1971.

60. FORTUIN N.J., HOOD W.P., CRAIGE E.: Evaluation of left ventricular function by echocardiography, *Circulation*, **46**:26, 1972.

61. FRAKER T.D., HARRIS P.J., BEHAR V.S., KISSLO J.A.: Detection and exclusion of interatrial shunts by two dimensional echocardiography and peripheral venous injection, *Circulation*, **59**:379, 1979.

62. FRENCH J.W., BAUM D., POPP R.L.: Echocardiographic findings in Uhl's anomaly, *Am. J. Cardiol.*, **36**:349, 1975.

63. FRENCH J.W., POPP R.: Variability of echocardiographic discontinuity in double outlet right ventricle and truncus arteriosus, *Circulation*, **51**:848, 1975.

64. GAASCH W.H.: Left ventricular radius to wall thickness ratio, *Am. J. Cardiol.*, **43**:1189, 1979.

65. GAGNE S., LAURENCEAU J.L., DUMESNIL J.G.: La physiologie particulière du septum interventriculaire dans la contraction cardiaque, *Ann. Cardiol. Angeiol.*, **25**:433, 1976.

66. GEHRKE J., LEEMAN S., RAPHAEL M. et al: Non invasive left ventricular volume determination by two dimensional echocardiography, *Brit. Heart. J.*, **37**:911, 1975.

67. GEWITZ M.H., WERNER J.C., KLEINMAN C.S. et al: Role of echocardiography in aortic stenosis: pre and postoperative studies, *Am. J. Cardiol.*, **43**:67, 1979.

68. GIBSON D.G.: Estimation of left ventricular size echocardiography, *Brit. Heart. J.*, **35**:128, 1973.

69. GIBSON T.C., GROSSMAN W., Mc LAURIN L.P. et al: An echocardiographic study of the interventricular septum in constrictive pericarditis, *Brit Heart. J.*, **38**:738, 1976.

70. GILBERT B.W., SCHATZ R.A., VON RAMM O.T. et al: Mitral valve prolapse: two dimensional echocardiographic and angiographic correlation, *Circulation*, **54**:716, 1976.

71. GOLDBERG B.B.: Suprasternal ultrasonography, *J.A.M.A.*, **215**:245, 1971.

72. GOLDBERG B.B.: Ultrasonic measurement of the aortic arch, right pulmonary artery and left atrium, *Radiology*, **101**:383, 1971.

73. GOLDMAN D.E., HUETER T.F.: Tabular data of the velocity and absorption of high frequency sound in mammalian tissue, *J. Acoust. Soc. Am.*, **28**:35, 1956.

74. GOODMAN M.J., THAM P., LANGFORD-KIDD B.S.: Echocardiography in the evaluation of the cyanotic newborn infant, *Br. Heart. J.*, **36**:154, 1974.

75. GRAMIAK R., SHAH P.M., KRAMER D.H.: Ultrasound cardiography: contrast studies in anatomy and function, *Radiology*, **92**:939, 1969.

76. GRAMIAK R., SHAH P.M.:Echocardiography of the normal and disead aortic valve, *Radiology*, **96**:1, 1970.

77. GRAMIAK R., SHAH P.M.: Cardiac ultrasonography a review of current applications., *Radiol. Clin. North. Am.*, **39**:469, 1971.

78. GRAMIAK R., KUNG K.J., NANDA N. et al: Echocardiographic diagnosis of transposition of the great vessels, *Radiology*, **106**:487, 1973.

79. GRIFFITH J.M., HENRY W.L.: A sector scanner for real time two dimensional echocardiography, *Circulation*, **49**:1147, 1974.

80. GROSSMAN W., JONES D., Mc LAURIN L.P.: Wall stress and patterns of hypertrophy in the human left ventricle, *J. Clin. Invest.*, **56**:56, 1975.

81. GUTGESELL H.P., PAQUET M., DUFF D.F. et al: Evaluation of left ventricular size and function by echocardiography. Results in normal children, *Circulation*, **56**:457, 1977.

82. HAEGLER D.J., TAJIK A.J., SEWARD J.B. et al: Further echocardiographic observations in atrio ventricular canal defect, *Circulation*, **52**:(suppl. II), 193, 1975 (abst).

83. HAEGLER D.J.: The utilisation of echocardiography in the differential diagnosis of cyanosis in the neonate, *Mayo. Clin. Proc.*, **51**:143, 1976.

84. HAEGLER D.J., TAJIK A.J., SEWARD J.B. et al: Real time wide angle sector echocardiography: atrio ventricular canal defect, *Circulation*, **59**:140, 1979.

85. HAEGLER D.J., TAJIK A.J., SEWARD J.B. et al: Wide angle two dimensional echocardiographic criterie for ventricular morphology, *Am. J. Cardiol.*, **45**:466, 1980 (abst).

86. HAGAN A.D., FRANCIS G.S., SAHN D.J. et al: Ultrasound evaluation of systolic anterior septal motion in patients with and without right ventricular volume overload, *Circulation*, **50**:248, 1974.

87. HENRY W.L., CLARK D.E., EPSTEIN S.E.: Assymetric septal hypertrophy; echocardiographic identification of he pathognomomic anatomic abnormality of I.H.S.S., *Circulation*, **47**:225, 1973.

88. HENRY W.L., MARON B.J., GRIFFITH J.L. et al: Differential diagnosis of abnormalies of the great arteries by real time two dimensional echocardiography, *Circulation*, **51**:283, 1975.

89. HENRY W.L., GRIFFITH J.M., MICHAELIS L.L. et al: Measurement of mitral orifice area in patients with mitral valve disease by real time, two dimensional echocardiography, *Circulation*, **51**:827, 1975.

90. HIRATA T., WOLFE S.B., POPP R.L. et al: Estimation of left atrial size using ultrasound, *Amer. Heart. J.*, **78**:43, 1969.

91. HIRSCHFELD S. , MEYER R.A., SCHWARTZ D.C. et al: Measurement of right and left ventricular systolic time intervals by echocardiography, *Circulation*, **51**:304, 1975.

92. HIRSCHFELD S. , MEYER R.A., SCHWARTZ D.C. et al: Echocardiographic assessment of pulmonary artery and pulmonary vascular resistance, *Circulation*, **52**:642, 1975.

93. HIRSHLEIFER J., CRAWFORD M., O'ROUKE R.A. et al: Influence of acute alterations in heart rate and systemic arterial pressure on echocardiographic measures of left ventricle heart performance in normal human subject, *Circulation*, **52**:835, 1975.

94. HOWRY D.H., BLISS W.R.: Ultrasonic visualization of soft tissue structures of the body, *J. Lab. Clin. Med.* **40**:579, 1952.

95. JOHNSON S.L., BAKER D.W., LUTE R.A. et al: Doppler echocardiography: The localization of cardiac murmurs, *Circulation*, **48**:810, 1973.

96. JOHNSON S.L., BAKER D.W.: Doppler echocardiography in KING D.L., Editor. Diagnostic ultrasound, *CV Mosby, Saint-Louis*, 1974.

97. JOYNER C.R., REID J.M., BOND J.P.: Reflected ultrasound in the assessment of mitral valve disease, *Circulation*, **27**:506, 1963.

98. JUGDUTT B.I., LEE S.J., Mc FARLANE D.: Non invasive assessment of left ventricular function from the mitral valve echogram; relation of final anterior mitral leafler closing velocity to peack dp/dt and aortic velocity, *Circulation*, **56**:861, 1978.

99. KALMANSON D., VEYRAT C., DERAI C. et al.: Non invasive technique for diagnosing atrial septal defect and assessing shunt volume using directional doppler ultrasound. Correlations with phasic flow velocity patterns of the shunt, *Brit. Heart. J.*, **34**:981, 1972.

100. KALMANSON D., VEYRAT C., BERNIER A. et al.: Diagnosis and evaluation of mitral valve disease using transeptal doppler ultrasound catherization, *Brit. Heart. J.*, **37**:257, 1975.

101. KASPER W., MEINERTZ T., KERSTING F.: Echocardiography in assessing acute pulmonary hypertension due to pulmonary embolism, *Am. J. Cardiol.*, **45**:567, 1980.

102. KEIDEL W.D.: Uber eine Methode zur Repiestrierig der Volumanderungen des Herzens am Menschen, *2. Z. Kreisl. Forch.*, **39**:257, 1950.

103. KIND D.L., STEEG C.N., ELLIS K.: Demonstration of transposition of the great arteries by cardiac ultrasonography, *Radiology*, **107**:181, 1973.

104. KISSLO J., VON RAMM O.T., FURSTONE F.: Cardiac imaging using a phased array ultrasound system II. Clinical technique and application, *Circulation*, **53**:262, 1976.

105. KOTLER M.N., SEGAL B.L., PARRY W.R.: Echocardiographic and phonocardiographic correlation of heart sounds and murmurs in KOTLER M.N., SEGAL B.L., Editors, Clinical Echocardiography - Cardiovascular Clinics, *F.A. Davis, Philadelphia*, 1978.

106. KRAUNZ R.F., RYAN T.J.: Ultrasound measurements of ventricular wall motion following administration of vasoactive drugs, *Am. J. Cardiol.*, **27**:464, 1971.

107. KRONIK G., SLANY J., MÖSSLACHER H.: Comparative value of eight M. Mode echocardiographic formulas for determining left ventricular stroke volume. A correlative study with thermo dilution and left ventricular single plane cineangiography, *Circulation*, **60**:1308, 1979.

108. KRONZON I., DANILOWICZ D., SCHLOSS M. et al: Tricuspid atresia, *Chest.*, **68**:818, 1975.

109. KRUEGER S.K., HOFSCHIRE P.J., FORKER A.D.: Echocardiography features of combined hypertrophic and membranous subvalvular aortic stenosis: a case report, *J. Clin. Ultrasound*, **4**:31, 1976.

110. KRUEGER S.K., FRENCH J.W., FORKER A.D. et al: Echocardiography in discrete subaortic stenosis, *Circulation*, **59**:506, 1979.

111. LACORTE M.A., HARADA K., WILLIAMS R.G.: Echocardiographic features of congenital left ventricular in flow obstruction, *Circulation*, **54**:562, 1976.

112. LACORTE M.A., FELLOWS K.E., WILLIAMS R.G.: Overriding tricuspid valve: echocardiographic and angiographic features, *Am. J. Cardiol.*, **37**:911, 1976.

113. LAIKEN S.L., JOHNSON A.D., BHARGAVA V. et al: Instantaneous transmitral blood flow and anterior mitral leaflet motion in man, *Circulation*, **59**:492, 1979.

114. LANGE L., SAHN D.J., ALLEW H. et al: Cross-sectional echocardiographic diagnosis of hypoplastic left heart syndrome, *Circulation*, **58**: (suppl. II) 50, 1978 (abst).

115. LANGEVIN M.P.: Les ondes ultrasonores, *Rev. Gén. Elect.*, **23**:626, 1928.

116. LAURENCEAU J.L., GUAY J.M., GAGNE S.: Echocardiography in the diagnosis of subaortic membranous sterosis, *Circulation*, **48**: (suppl. III) 46, 1973 (abst).

117. LAURENCEAU J.L., DELISLE G., GUAY J.L. et al: Etude des tétralogies de Fallot par échocardiographie, *Arch. Mal. Cœur*, **68**:505, 1975.

118. LAURENCEAU J.L., DUMESNIL J.G.: Right and left ventricular dimensions as determinants of ventricular septal motion, *Chest.* **69**:388, 1976.

119. LAURENCEAU J.L., DUMESNIL J.G.: Fonction ventriculaire globale (une analyse de l'échocardiogramme), *Un. Med. Can.*, **106**:172, 1977.

120. LAURENCEAU J.L., LIEHNART J.F., MALERGUE M.C. et al: Données échocardiographiques dans le syndrome du ventricule droit papyracé, *Arch. Mal. Cœur*, **72**:258, 1979.

121. bis LAURENCEAU J.L., MALERGUE M.C.: Intérêt de l'échocardiographie dans les urgences cardiovasculaires (en dehors des cardiopathies congénitales), *Arch. Mal. Cœur*, **72**:924, 1979.

121. LAYTON C., GENT G., PRIDIE R. et al: Diastolic closure rate of normal mitral valve, *Brit. Heart. J.*, **35**:1066, 1973.

122. LELE P.P.: Applications of ultrasound in medecine, *N. Engl. J. Med.*, **286**:1317, 1972.

123. LEWIS A.B., TAKAHASHI M.: Echocardiographic assessment of left to right shunt volume in children with ventricular septal defect, *Circulation*, **54**:78, 1976.

124. LIEPPE W., BEHAR V.S., SCALLON R.V.: Detection of tricuspid regurgitation with two dimensional echocardiography and peripheral vein injections, *Circulation*, **57**:128, 1978.

125. LINHART J.W., MINTZ G.S., SEGAL B.L. et al: left ventricular volume measurement by echocardiography: Fact or fiction? *Am. J. Cardiol.*, **36**:114, 1975.

126. LINTERMANS J.: Deductive echocardiographic diagnosis in congenital heart disease. Lancee C.T. Editor. Echocardiology. MARTINIUS NIJHOFF Publishers, *the Hague*, 1979.

127. LUNDSTRÖM N.R.: Ultrasound cardiographic studies of the mitral valve region in young infants with mitral atresia, mitral stenosis, hypoplasia of the left ventricle, and cor triatriatum, *Circulation*, **45**:324, 1972.

128. LUNDSTRÖM N.R.: Echocardiography in the diagnosis of Ebstein's anomaly of the tricuspid valve, *Circulation*, **47**:597, 1973.

129. Mc DONALD I.G.: Echocardiographic demonstration of abnormal motion of the interventricular septum in left sundle branch block, *Circulation*, **48**:272, 1973.

143

130. MALERGUE M.C., LAURENCEAU J.L., DUMESNIL J.G. et al: Echocardiographie: valves auriculo-ventriculaires normales et pathologiques, *Un. Med. Can.*, **106**:159, 1977.

131. MALERGUE M.C., LAURENCEAU J.L., DUMESNIL J.G.: Echocardiographic: valves aortique et pulmonaire normales et pathologiques, *Un. Med. Can.*, **106**:166, 1977.

132. MARTIN M.A., FIELLER N.R.J.: Echocardiography in cardiovascular drug assessment, *Brit. Heart. J.*, **41**:536, 1979.

133. MARTIN R.P., RAKOWSKI H., KLEIMAN J.H. et al: Reliability and reproductibility of two dimensionnal echocardiographic measurement of the stenotic mitral valve orifice area, *Am. J. Cardiol.*, **43**:560, 1979.

134. MEHTA S., HIRSCHFIELD S., RIGGS T. et al: Echocardiographic estimation of ventricular hypoplasia in complete atrio-ventricular canal, *Circulation*, **59**:888, 1979.

135. MEYER R.A., KAPLAN S.: Echocardiography in the diagnosis of hypoplasia of the left or right ventricles in the neonate, *Circulation*, **46**:55, 1972.

136. MEYER R.A., KAPLAN S.: Non invasive technics in pediatric cardiovascular disease, *Prog. Cardiovasc. DIS*, **15**:341, 1973.

137. MILLS P., MOOS S., CRAIGE E.: Simultaneous dual echocardiography. A new technique for investigating valvular, ventricular and acoustic events, *Circulation*, **54**:(sup. II) 62, 1976 (abst.).

138. MILNER S., MEYER R.A., VENABLES A.W. et al: Mitral and tricuspid valve closure in congenital heart disease, *Circulation*, **54**:513, 1976.

139. MINTZ G.S., KOTLER M.N., SEGAL B.L. et al: Two dimensional echographic recognition of the descending thoracic aorta, *Am. J. Cardiol.*, **44**:232, 1979.

140. MIRRO M.J., ROGER E.W., WEYMAN A.E. et al: Angular displacement of the papillary muscles during the cardiac cycle, *Circulation*, **60**:327, 1979.

141. MURRAY J.A., JOHNSTON W., REID J.M.: Echocardiographic determination of left ventricular dimensions, volumes and performance, *Am. J. Cardiol.*, **30**:252, 1972.

142. NADAS A.S., FYLER D.C.: Pediatric Cardiology (3rd edition), *Philadelphia Sanders*, 1972.

143. NANDA N.C., GRAMIAK R., MANNING J.A. et al: Echocardiographic recognition of the congenital bicuspid aortic valve, *Circulation*, **49**:870, 1974.

144. NANDA N.C., GRAMIAK R., MANNING J.A.: Echocardiographic studies of the tricuspid valve in atrial septal defect, *Circulation*, (suppl. III) **50**:236, 1974.

145. NANDA N.C., GRAMIAK R., ROBINSON T.I. et al: Echocardiography evaluation of pulmonary hypertension, *Circulation*, **50**:575, 1974.

146. NANDA N.C., GRAMIAK R., MANNING J.A.: Echocardiography of the tricuspid valve in congenital left ventricular-right atrial communication, *Circulation*, **51**:268, 1975.

147. NANDA N.C., GRAMIAK R., MANNING J.A. et al: Echocardiographic features of subpulmonic obstruction in dextro-transposition of the great vessels, *Circulation*, **51**:515, 1975.

148. NANDA N.C., STEWART S., GRAMIAK R. et al: Echocardiography of the intra-atrial baffle in dextro-transposition of the great vessels, *Circulation*, **51**:1130, 1975.

149. NANDA N.C., GRAMIAK R., MANNING J.A. et al: Echocardiographic identification of the interatrial septum: Clinical usefulness, *Circulation*, (suppl. II) **52**:221, 1975 (abst.).

150. ORSMOND G.S., RUTTENBERG H.D., BESSINGER F.B. et al: Echocardiographic features of total anomalous pulmonary venous connection to the coronary sinus, *Am. J. Cardiol.*, **41**:597, 1978.

151. PAQUET M., GUTGESELL H.: Echocardiographic features of total anomalous pulmonary venous connection, *Circulation*, **51**:599, 1975.

152. PARAKOS J.A., GROSSMAN W., SALTZ S. et al: A non invasive technique for the determination of velocity of circumferential fiber shortening in man, **29**:610, 1971.

153. PAULSEN W.J., BOUGHNER D.R., FRIESEN A., PERSAUD J.A.: Ventricular response to isometric and isotonic exercise: Echocardiographic assessment, *Brit. Heart. J.*, **42**:521, 1979.

154. PAYVANDI M.N., KERBER R.E.: Echocardiography in congenital and acquired absence of the pericardium: an echocardiographic mimic of right ventricular volume overload, *Circulation*, **53**:86, 1976.

155. PERNOD J., SERVELLE M., HAGUENAUER G. et al: Correlations entre échocardiographie par ultrasons et constatations anatomochirurgicales dans les cardiopathies mitrales (à propos de 140 corrélations), *Arch. Mal. Cœur*, **66**:333, 1973.

144

156. PERNOD J., KERMAREC J., RICHARD D. et al: Détermination de la contractibilité myocardique par échographie ultrasonique, *Nouv. Presse Méd.*, **4**:1113, 1975.

157. PIERONI D.R., HOMCY E., FREEDOM R.M.: Echocardiography in atrioventricular canal defect: a clinical spectrum, *Am. J. Cardiol.*, **35**:54, 1975.

158. POCOSKI D.J., SHAH P.L.: Physiologic correlates of echocardiographic pulmonary valve motion in diastole, *Circulation*, **58**:1064, 1978.

159. POHOST G.M., DINSMORE R.E., RUBINSTEIN J.J. et al: The echocardiogram of the anterior leaflet of the mitral valve: Correlation with hemodynamic and cineroentgenographic studies in dogs, *Circulation*, **51**:88, 1975.

159. bis POMBO J.F., TROY B.L., RUSSEL R.O.: Left ventricular volumes and ejection fraction by echocardiography, *Circulation*, **43**:480, 1971.

160. POPP R.L. WOLFE S.B., HIRATA T. et al: Estimation of right and left ventricular size by ultrasound. A study of the echoes from the interventricular septum, *Am. J. Cardiol.*, **24**:523, 1969.

161. PORTS T.A., SILVERMAM N.H., SCHILLER N.B.: Two dimensional echocardiographic assessment of Ebstein's anomaly, *Circulation*, **58**:336, 1978.

162. PRASQUIER R., BARTHELEMY M., VERLIN P. et al : Echocardiographie bidimensionnelle dans l'infarctus aigu du myocarde, *Arch. Mal. Cœur.*, **72**:1069, 1979.

163. RADFORD D.J., BLUM K.J., IZUKAWA T. et al: Echocardiographic assessment of bicuspid aortic valve. Angiographic and pathological correlates, *Circulation*, **53**:80, 1976.

164. REPORT of the Inter-Society Commission for heart disease resources: Optimal resources for ultrasonic examination of the heart, *Circulation*, **51 A-I**, 1975.

165. ROELANDT J., VAN DORP W.G., BOMIN et al: Resolution problems in echocardiology: a source of interpretation errors, *Am. J. Cardiol.*, **37**:256, 1976.

166. ROGE C.L., SILVERMAN N.H., HART P.A. et al: Cardiac structure growth pattern determined by echocardiography, *Circulation*, **57**:285, 1978.

167. ROGE C.L., SNIDER R., SILVERMAN N.H.: Echocardiographic evaluation of left ventricular in flow obstruction in children using an 80° two dimensional sector scanner. In Lancee C.T. Editor Echocardiology MARTINIUS NIJHOFF, *the Hague*, 1979.

168. ROTHBAUM D.A., DILLON J.C., CHANG S. et al: Echocardiographic manifestations of right sinus of valsalva arreuysms, *Circulation*, **49**:768,1974.

169. RUBINSTEIN J.J., POHOST G.M., DINSMORE R.E. et al: The echocardiographic determination of mitral valve opening and closure; correlation with hemodynamic studies in man, *Circulation*, **51**:98, 1975.

170. SAHN D.J., TERRY R., O'ROURKE R. et al: Multiple crystal cross-sectional echocardiography in the diagnosis of cyanotic congenital heart, *Circulation*, **50**:230, 1974.

171. SAHN D.J., VAUCHER Y., WILLIAMS D.F. et al: Echocardiographic detection of large left to right shunts and cardionyopathies in infants and children, *Am. J. Cardiol.*, **38**:73, 1976.

172. SAHN D.J., ALLEN H.D., Mc DONALD G. et al: Real time cross-sectional echocardiographic diagnosis of coarctation of the aorta, *Circulation*, **56**:762, 1977.

173. SAHN D.J., ALLEN H.D.: Real time cross sectional echocardiographic imaging and measurement of the patent ductus arteriosus in infants and children, *Circulation*, **58**:343, 1978.

174. SAHN D.J., DEMARIA A., KISSLO J., WEYMAN A.: — The committee on M Mode standardization of the american society echocardiography. Recommandations regarding quantification in M Mode echocardiography: results of a survey of echocardiographic measurements, *Circulation*, **58**:1072, 1978.

175. SAHN D.J., ALLEN H.D., LANGE L.W. et al: Cross-sectional echocardiographic diagnosis of the sites of total anomalous pulmonary venous drainage, *Circulation*, **60**:1317, 1979.

176. SAPIRE T.W., BLACK I.F.S.: Echocardiographic detection of aneurysm of the interventricular septum associated with ventricular septal defect, *Am. J. Cardiol.*, **36**:797, 1975.

177. SCHILLER N.B., SILVERMAN N.H,: Two dimensional ultrasonic cardiac imaging in KLEID J.J. Editor. Echocardiography interpretation and diagnosis, *Appleton-Century-Crofts, New York*, 1978.

178. SCHILLER N.B.: Echocardiography of the right ventricular outflow tract and adjoining structures: In KLEID J.J. Editor. Echocardiography interpretation diagnosis, *Appleton-Century-Crofts, New York*, 1978.

179. SCHILLER N.B., ACQUATELLA H., PORTS T.A. et al: Left ventricular volume for paired biplane two dimensional echocardiography, *Circulation*, **60**:547, 1979.

180. SEWARD J.B., TAJIK A.J., SPANGLER J.G. et al: Echocardiographic contrast studies: initial experience, *Mayo. Clin. Proc.*, **50**:163, 1975.

181. SEWARD J.B., TAJIK A.J., RITTER D.G.: Echocardiographic features of straddling tricuspid valve, *Mayo. Clin. Proc.*, **50**:427, 1975.

182. SEWARD J.B., TAJIK A.J., HAGLER D.J. et al: Peripheral venous contrast echocardiography, *Am. J. Cardiol.*, **339**:202, 1977.

183. SEWARD J.B., TAJIK A.J., HAGLER D.J. et al: Echocardiogram in common (single) ventricle: angiographic-anatomic correlation, *Am. J. Cardiol.*, **39**:217, 1977.

184. SEWARD J.B., TAJIK A.J., HAGLER D.J. et al: Contrast echocardiography in single or common ventricle, *Circulation*, **55**:513, 1977.

185. SEWARD J.B., TAJIK A.J.: Current status of echocardiography in cyanotic congenital heart diseases in KOTLER M.N., SEGAL B.L. Editors, Clinical Echocardiography. Cardiovascular Clinics. *F.A. Davis, Philadelphia*, 1978.

186. SEWARD J.B., TAJIK A.J.: Echocardiographic spectrum of tricuspid atresia, *Mayo. Clin. Proc.*, **53**:100, 1978.

187. SILVERMAN N.H., LEWIS A.B., HEIMANN M.A. et al: Echocardiographic assessment of ductus arteriosus shunt in premature infants, *Circulation*, **50**:821, 1974.

188. SILVERMAN N.H., SCHILLER N.B.: Apex Echocardiography: a two dimensional technique for evaluating congenital heart disease, *Circulation*, **57**:503, 1978.

189. SJÖGREN A.L.: Left ventricular wall thickness determined by ultrasound in 100 subjects without heart disease, *Chest.*, **60**:341, 1971.

190. SNIDER A.R., PORTS T.A., SILVERMAN N.H.: Venous anomalies of the coronary sinus: detection by M Mode, two dimensional and contrast echocardiography, *Circulation*, **60**:721, 1979.

191. SOLINGER R., ELBL F., MINHAS K.: Echocardiography in the normal neonate, *Circulation*, **47**:108, 1973.

192. SOLINGER R., ELBL F., MINHAS K.: Echocardiographic features of complete transposition of great vessels in infancy, *Am. J. Cardiol.*, **31**:158, 1973.

193. SOLINGER R., ELBL F., MINHAS K.: Deductive echocardiographic analysis in infants with congenital heart disease, *Circulation*, **50**:1072, 1974.

194. STARLIN M.R., CRAWFORD M.H., O'ROURKE R.A. et al: Acurracy of sub-xiphoid echocardiography for assessing left ventricular size and performance, *Circulation*, **61**:367, 1980.

195. STEFADOUROS M.A., DOUGHERTY M.S., GROSSMAN W. et al: Determination of systemic vascular resistance by a non invasive technique, *Circulation*, **47**:101, 1973.

196. STRUNK B.L., LONDON E.J., FITZGERALD J. et al: The assessment of mitral stenosis and prosthetic mitral valve obstruction, using the posterior aortic wall echocardiogram, *Circulation*, **55**:885, 1977.

197. TAJIK A.J., GAU G.T., RITTER D.G. et al: Echocardiographic pattern of right ventricular diastolic volume overload in children, *Circulation*, **46**:36, 1972.

198. TAJIK A.J., GAU G.T., GIULIANI E.R. et al: Echocardiogram in Ebstein's anomaly with Wolff-Parkinson. White preexitation syndrome, type B., *Circulation*, **47**:813, 1973.

199. TAJIK A.J., SEWARD J.B.: Contrast echocardiography in KOTLER M.N., SEGAL B.L. Editors, Clinical Echocardiography Cardiovascular clinics, *F.A. Davis, Philadelphia*, 1978.

200. TAJIK A.J., SEWARD J.B., HAGLER D.J. et al: Two dimensional real time ultrasonic imaging of the heart and great vessels, *Mayo. Clin. Proc.*, **53**:271, 1978.

201. TEI C., TANAKA H., KASHIMA T. et al: Echocardiographic analysis of interatrial septal motion, *Am. J. Cardiol.*, **44**:472, 1979.

202. TEICHHOLZ L.E., COHEN M.V., SONNENBLICK E.H. et al: Study of left ventricular geometry and function by B-Scan ultrasonography in patients with and without asynergy, *New. Engl. J. Med.*, **291**:1220, 1974.

203. TEICHHOLZ L.E., KREULEN T., HERMAN M.V. et al: Problems in echocardiographic volume determinations: echocardiographic-angiographic correlations in the presence or absence of asynergy, *Am. J. Cardiol*, **37**:7, 1976.

204. TRAILL T.A., GIBSON D.G., BROWN D.J.: Study of left ventricular left thickness and dimension changes using echocardiography, *Brit. Heart. J.*, **40**:162, 1978.

205 TRICOT R., VEBER G., STOLTZ J.P.: L'echocardiographie: application et apport dans les cardiopathies mitrales, *Arch. Mal. Cœur*, **62**:1353, 1969.

206. TROY B.L., POMBO J., RACKLEY C.E.: Measurement of left ventricular wall thickness and mass by echocardiography, *Circulation*, **45**:602, 1972.

207. UEDA K., KUWAKI K., INONE K.: Three dimensional display and volume determination of the left ventricle by two dimensional echocardiography, *Am. J. Cardiol.*, **45**:471, 1980 (abstract).

208. UHL H.S.: Previously undescribed congenital malformation of the heart: Almost total absence of the myocardium of the right ventricle. *Bull. John Hopkins Hosp.*, **91**:197, 1952.

209. UPTON M.T., GIBSON D.G.: The study of left ventricular function from digitized echocardiograms, *Progr. Cardiovasc. DIS.*, **20**:359, 1978.

210. UPTON M.T., GIBSON D.G.: The study of left ventricular function from digitized echocardiograms., *Progr. Cardiovasc. DIS.*, **20**:359, 1978.

211. USHER B.W., GOULDEN D., MURGO J.P.: Echocardiographic detection of supravalvular aortic stenosis, *Circulation*, **49**:1257, 1974.

212. VAN MEURS-VANWOEZIK H., KLEIN H.W., KREDIET P.: Normal internal calibers of ostia of great arteries and of aortic isthmus in infants and children, *Brit. Heart. J.*, **39**:860, 1977.

213. VAN PRAAGH R., VAN PRAAGH S., VLAD P. et al: Anatomic types of congenital dextrocardia: diagnosis and embryologic implications. *Am. J. Cardiol.*, **13**:510, 1964.

214. VAN PRAAGH R., VAN PRAAGH S., VLAD P. et al: Diagnosis of the anatomic types of single or common ventricles, *Am. J. Cardiol.*, **15**:345, 1965.

215. VAN PRAAGH R., VAN PRAAGH S.: Isolated ventricular inversion. A consideration of the morphogenesis, definition and diagnosis of non-transposed and transposed great arteries., *Am. J. Cardiol.*, **17**:395, 1966.

216. VAN PRAAGH R., VAN PRAAGH S., NEBESAR R.A. et al: Tetralogy of Fallot: under development of the pulmonary infundibulum and its sequelae, *Am. J. Cardiol.*, **26**:25, 1970.

217. VAN PRAAGH R., WEINBERG R., VAN PRAAGH S.: Malposition of the heart. In heart disease in infants, children and adolescents. 2nd ed. edited by MOSS. A.S., ADAMS F.M., EMMANOUILIDES G.C., WILLIAMS AND WILKINS., *Baltimore*, 1978.

218. VIGNOLA P.A., WALKER H.J., GOLD H.K. et al: Alteration of the left ventricular pressure-volume relationships in man and its effect of the mitral echocardiographic diastolic closure slope, *Circulation*, **56**:586, 1977.

219. VICK G.W., SERWER G.A.: Echocardiographic evaluation of the post-operative tetralogy of Fallot patient, *Circulation*, **58**:842, 1978.

220. VON RAMM O.T., THURSTONE F.L.: Cardiac imaging using a phased array ultrasound system, *Circulation*, **53**:258, 1976.

221. WAAG R.C., GRAMIAK R.: Ultrasound Basics in GRAMMIAK R. and WAAG R.C., Editors, Cardiac ultrasound, 2CV Mosby Saint-Louis, 1975.

222. WANN L.S., WEYMAN A.E., DILLON J.C. et al: Premature pulmonary valve opening, *Circulation*, **55**:128, 1977.

223. WEYMAN A.E., DILLON J.C., FEIGENBAUM H. et al: Echocardiographic patterns of pulmonic valve motion in valvular pulmonic stenosis, *Am. J. Cardiol.*, **34**:644, 1974.

224. WEYMAN A.E., DILLON J.C., FEIGENBAUM H. et al: Echocardiographic patterns of pulmonic valve motion with pulmonary hypertension, *Circulation*, **50**:905, 1974.

225. WEYMAN A.E., DILLON J.C., FEIGENBAUM H. et al: Echocardiographic differentiation of infundibular from valvular pulmonary stenosis, *Am. J. Cardiol.*, **36**:21, 1975.

226. WEYMAN A.E., FEIGENBAUM H., DILLON J.C. et al: Cross-sectional echocardiography in assessing the severity of valvular aortic stenosis, *Circulation*, **52**:828, 1975.

227. WEYMAN A.E., FEIGENBAUM H., DILLON J.C. et al: Cross-sectional echocardiography in evaluating patients with discrete subaortic stenosis, *Am. J. Cardiol.*, **37**:358, 1976.

228. WEYMAN A.E., FEIGENBAUM H., DILLON J.C. et al: Non invasive visualization of the left main coronary artery by cross-sectional echocardiography, *Circulation*, **54**:169, 1976.

229. WEYMAN A.E.: Pulmonary valve echo motion in clinical practice, *Am. J. Medecine*, **62**:843, 1977.

230. WEYMAN A.E., HURWITZ R.A., GIROD D.A. et al: Cross-sectional echocardiographic visualization of the stenotic pulmonary valve, *Circulation*, **56**:769, 1977.

231. WEYMAN A.E., CALDWELL R.L., HÜRWITZ R.A. et al: Cross-sectional echocardiographic caracterization of aortic obstruction: I. Supravalvular aortic stenosis and aortic hypoplasia, *Circulation*, **57**:491, 1978.

232. WEYMAN A.E., CALDWELL R.L., HÜRWITZ R.A. et al: Cross-sectional echocardiographic detection of aortic obstruction: II. Coarctation of the aorta, *Circulation*, **57**:498, 1978.

233. WEYMAN A.E., WANN L.S., CALDWELL R.L. et al: Negative contrast echocardiography: a new method for detecting left to right shunts, *Circulation*, **59**:498, 1979.

234. WILD J.J., NEAL D.: Use of high frequency ultrasonic waves for detecting changes in texture in living tissues, *Lancet 1:* **655,** 1951.

235. WILLIAMS R.G.: Echocardiographic features of left ventricular out flow obstruction in transposition of the great arteries, *Pediatr. Rev.*, **8**:355, 1974.

236. WILLIAMS R.G., RUDD M.: Echocardiographic features of endocardial cushion defect, *Circulation*, **49**:418, 1974.

237. WILLIAMS R.G., TUCKER C.R.: Echocardiographic diagnosis of congenital heart disease, *Little, Brown and Company. Boston*, 1977.

238. WINTERS W.L., GIMENEZ J.L., SOLOFF L.: Clinical applications of ultrasound the analysis of prosthetic ball valve function, *Am. J. Cardiol.* , **19**:97, 1967.

239. YEH H.C., WINSBERG F., MERGER E.M.: Echocardiographic aortic valve orifice dimension: Its use in evaluation aortic stenosis and cardiac output, *J. Clin. Ultrasound*, **1**:182, 1973.

240. YEH H.C., STEINFELD L., BARON M.: Echocardiography of double outlet right ventricle. A new diagnostic criteria, *Circulation*, **52**:(suppl. II) 120, 1975.

SUBJECT INDEX

TABLE OF PLATES

Achevé d'imprimer par l'Imprimerie Ch. Corlet, 14110 Condé-sur-Noireau

N° d'Imprimeur : 6719 — Dépôt légal : 1er trimestre 1981